365

SEX

POSITIONS

Published by:
AMORATA PRESS,
an imprint of Ulysses Press
PO Box 3440
Berkeley, CA 94703

ISBN13: 978-1-64604-033-9
Library of Congress Control Number: 2020931877

Printed in China through Printplus Ltd.

0 9 8 7 6 5 4

Acquisitions editor: Nick Denton-Brown
Managing editor: Claire Chun
Copyeditors: Lauren Harrison, Lily Chou
Proofreader: Barbara Schultz
Design and layout: Wade Nights
Photographs: Hollan Publishing, Inc.

365
SEX
POSITIONS

A New Way Every Day for a Steamy, Erotic Year

Lisa Sweet

Amorata Press

TRIBAL RHYTHM 1

He will love the full view and his ability
to control her every movement.

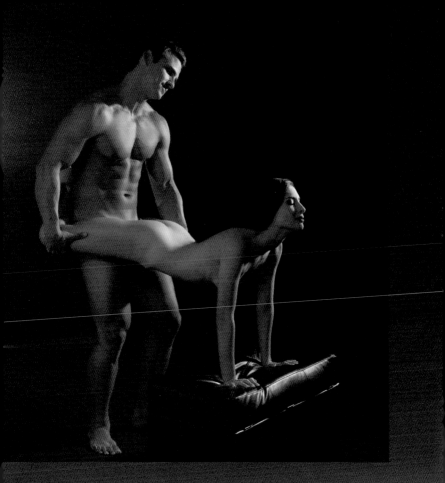

2 THE CHARIOT

Her pleasure is all in his hands. He lifts her gams higher to fiddle her diddle or lowers them to add a little slow-down pressure on his own bow.

CLIMB THE HILL 3

Reaching the heights of pleasure in this position is a bit of a high-wire act since the higher-than-usual placement of her hips can create some slippage before they can peak.

4 THE EDGE

All it takes to line up both partners' bits so that his every move rubs her in an oh-so-good way is a little furniture rearrangement that tilts her pelvis up and creates an exquisite, erotic, up-and-down motion.

PEEK-A-BOO 5

The only thing better than having him
tiptoe up behind her and slide one in
is for her to take a thrilling sneak peek
as they reach their passion peaks.

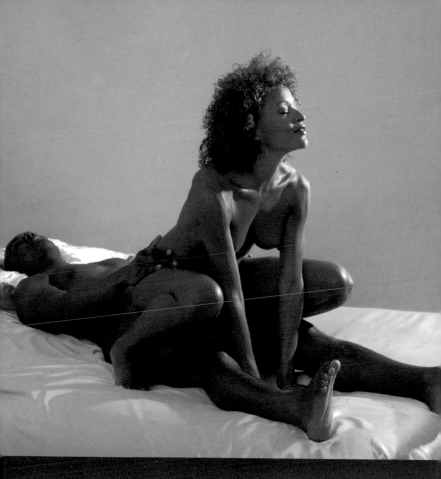

6 HAPPY TRAILS

This pose is all butt, legs, and hips — hers — which will make him very, very, very happy.

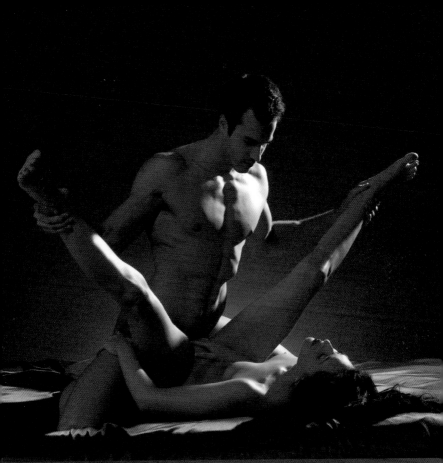

SPREAD EAGLE **7**

This is a very accommodating pose for him,
but with her legs held wide, she will lose out on
some of the friction of his thrusting, so giving
herself a helping hand should send her soaring.

8 THE CIRCUS

Twisting her back and forth in a jaw-dropping rotation will make both partners feel like sexual dynamos and may even keep them spinning for rounds two, three, and four!

RAPUNZEL 9

In this fairy tale position, the long-haired princess arches back so her tresses sway against the tingly, thin, nerve-rich skin on his thighs and ticklish toes.

10 CAT'S CRADLE

Using her feet to push him in and out and all about, this sneakily simple position allows her to guide his directional exactly where she wants it — nesting against all of her most sensitive spots.

THE HANDSTAND 11

An intense pose that's sure to blow him over. Just be careful his arms don't also go limp at the end or he will experience a most unwanted header.

12 THE WATCHER

Men are more visually stimulated than women. Lifting his leg gives him a good bird's-eye view of the action without giving up any of the pleasure.

BACK SHOW 13

Any position that gives him unlimited access to
her wiggling backside will motivate him to race
that extra mile she needs to cross her finish line.

14 LANGUID LEGS

Despite its visual pizzazz, this is actually an easy move to master, making it primo for some splendid rub-a-dub-dubs in all the right places — ecstasy without a lot of high-energy commitment.

CROUCHING TIGER 15

The more ferocious pressure she applies
to him with her mouth, the louder she
will get his dragon to roar. Beware of
shooting flames and sharp fangs.

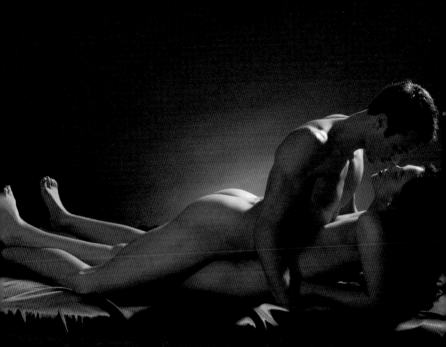

16 ELECTRIC SLIDE

A perfect position for creating some
extra friction between their bodies — just
watch out for carpet burns!

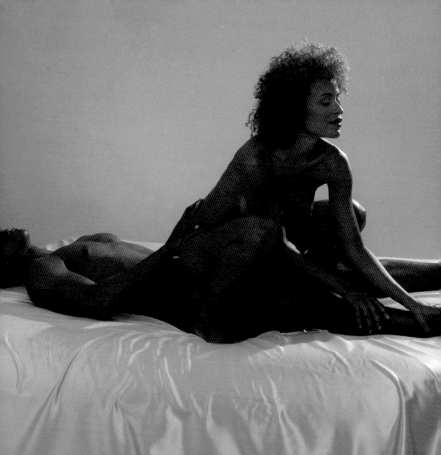

TWIST AND SHOUT 17

The key move here is for her to twist back and forth rather than up and down to gradually screw him in delectably deep and tight.

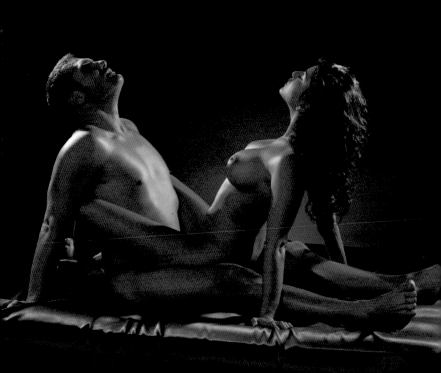

18 SEESAW

Lovers can divvy up the amorous action by grinding in tandem — one pushes up and forward as the other thrusts down and back. The teamwork will result in each gaining from the other's erotic efforts.

FREESTYLE 19

He can rock her side to side or up and down,
taking his cue from her — if she pushes her
body into him, she likes his angle; if she
pulls back, he should try something else.

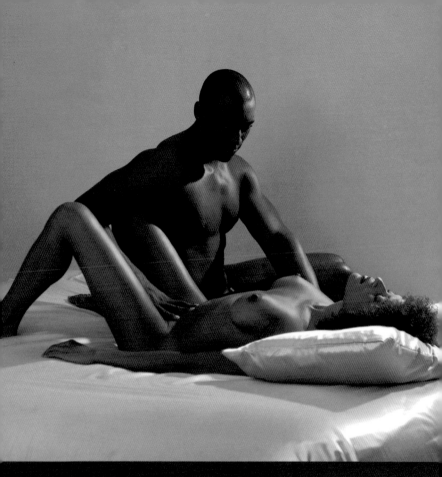

20 LADIES FIRST

Here's her opportunity for multiple orgasms by letting him focus entirely on her for the first round before they move on to mutual pleasuring.

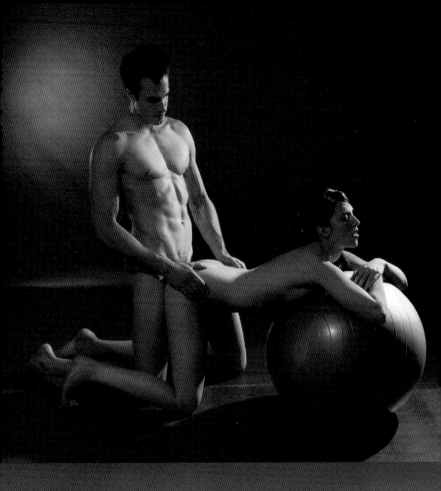

ROLLOVER 21

Roll up and over or back and down on the ball to find the perfect angle of penetration.

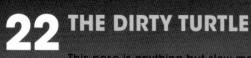

22 THE DIRTY TURTLE

This pose is anything but slow moving, as the sight of her bottom combined with the vibrations of her mouth will put him on the fast track to ecstasy.

THE CATAPULT **23**

She'll feel like he is sending her flying as he
pulls her up into the air, but the only thing that
will go rocketing in this pose is her bliss level.

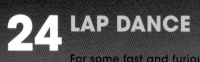

24 LAP DANCE

For some fast and furious fun, she can lower herself onto him and gyrate around in time to her own beat.

THE CLASSIC 25

This traditional oral favorite is tough to lick. While he's controlling the action, her hands can roam and caress the rest of his body to his spine-tingling delight.

26 THE BIG DIP

He can use the extra access provided by
the open edge of the bed to go in deep
while she can use her grounded leg to lift
up and meet him halfway, creating lots
of feel-fabulous friction down below.

POWER PUMPER 27

She gets to choose between shallow and deep
thrusting but she should perfect her posture and
keep a very straight back to avoid him popping
out of her like a disappointed jack-in-the-box.

28 GET A LEG OVER

If he's not hung like Moby Dick, she can open her legs wider and lift her top foot straight up in the air, making it easier for him to cross her threshold.

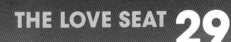

THE LOVE SEAT **29**

Unlike most female-superior poses, she won't
be taking him for a ride: Her balancing act
means that he'll end up doing most of the
thrusting, so she can sit back and concentrate
on how amazing his stroking feels.

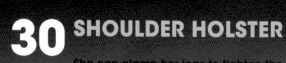

30 SHOULDER HOLSTER

She can clamp her legs to tighten the
sensations or widen them to give him an
excellent view of the action. Either way, she'll
be giving her G-spot a hot and sticky workout.

BALL GAME 31

This is a good pose for getting in some extra offside plays. Beyond tackling his tackle with her mouth, she can score an extra point by reaching in with her hand to fumble his balls.

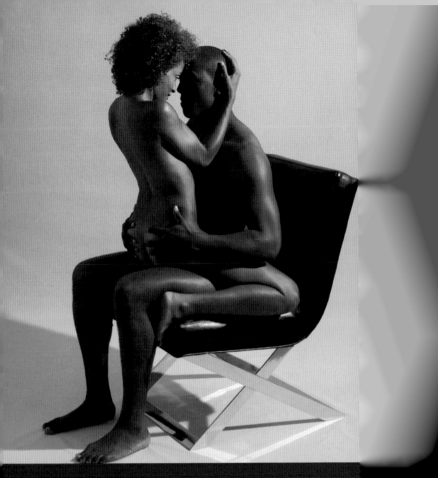

32 CLOSE ENCOUNTERS

Sitting seems like the least exciting way to g
whisked off your feet, but sweet surprise — it
actually perfect for when lovers are in the m
for some intimate, slow, romantic romping.

THE LOTUS 33

Crisscrossing her legs will help send their lovemaking to a higher spiritual plane that just happens to result in out-of-this-world-and-the-next orgasms.

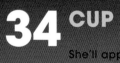

34 CUP

She'll appreciate the extra neck support
as he starts shaking his booty.

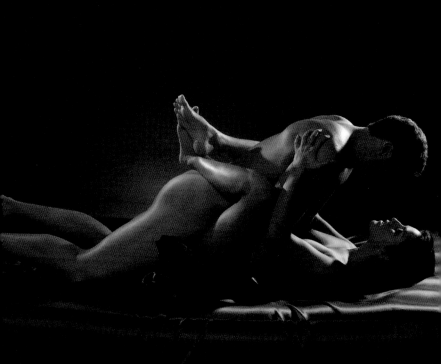

THE DEEP

The higher she raises her legs, the farther
he will penetrate her. What's more, she
can pull him deeper and deeper into her,
a smooth move that will soon have both
partners coming up, gasping for air.

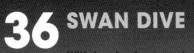

36 SWAN DIVE

With her body spanning his, he'll be completely
surrounded by her...and love every minute of it.

THE CRAZY CAT 37

The stronger he is, the higher her kitty
will climb in this gravity-defying twist on
the Coital Alignment Technique. All that
frontal friction on her purr spot means
that she will be meowing with pleasure.

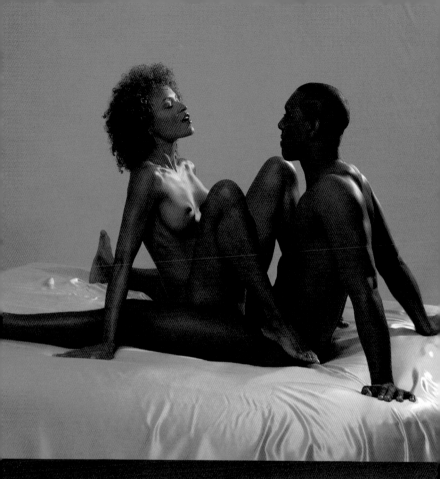

38 QUEEN FOR THE DAY

She can tease and please him with unexpected hip twists, including back-and-forth rubs, side-to-side shakes and up-and-down dynamo pumps. Not knowing what's coming next will keep him on the edge of his hot seat.

DAISY CHAIN 39

Take time to kiss, cuddle and caress each other before he reaches down and brings her to orgasm while she enjoys teasing him and feeling his excitement by rubbing back against him.

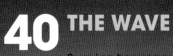

40 THE WAVE

Swaying her upper body from side to side
does more than make her look like an
enthusiastic sports fan — the extra sensations
it creates will turn his soft line drive into a
pulse-pounding, record-breaking home run.

SURPRISE PARTY 41

There's an enticing element of the unknown in this pose since both partners can easily work their hands into the mix, but neither can see which next naughty-nooky move the other is planning.

42 THE HAMMOCK

Few women can hold this advanced position since she'll need to have a strong neck or a background in gymnastics — or both.

BLASTOFF 43

When they want a really explosive
show, this position gives both partners
a great view of the fireworks.

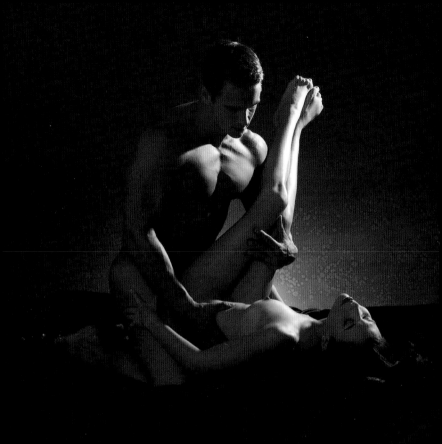

44 SEXY SAMBA

She can relax into his arms and concentrate
more on the lusty moves he is making
than maintaining her balance.

JUNGLE FEVER 45

Just being bent over is hot and primal, especially when they take the action outdoors. But when he grabs her hips and pushes himself in? Time for a Tarzan-meets-Jane howl.

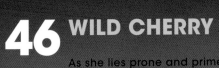

46 WILD CHERRY

As she lies prone and primed with her arms above her head, it's up to him to triple the trysting pleasure by kissing and caressing her all over with his hands or tongue.

THE CARNAL CHAISE 47

Supported by the backrest of a strong chair,
he can hold all her weight as she presses
against him and down into his lap.

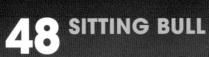

48 SITTING BULL

Easier than it looks. The nice thing about this
move is that it doesn't take a lot of effort to
get into position, but the sideways angle still
generates a lot of spine-tingling, sexy tension.

THE COW 49

In this superdeep position, she can contract and relax her pelvic muscles to milk him into a frothy shake (wait until after yoga class before trying this one).

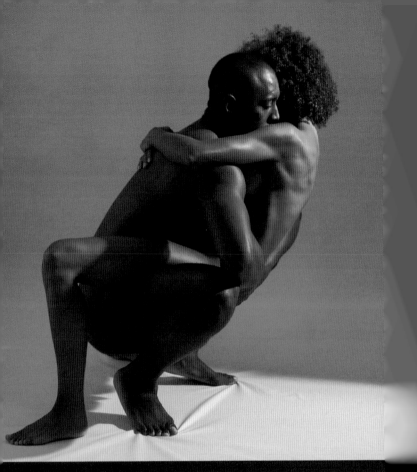

50 THE CROUCH SLOUCH

Despite the tricky balance, she gets to have a lot of control over the speed, angle, and motion here because she can use her arms and legs to help her maneuver.

THE FLAT BACK 51

This is a nice beginner position that lets him
stay in control of how deep his love goes.

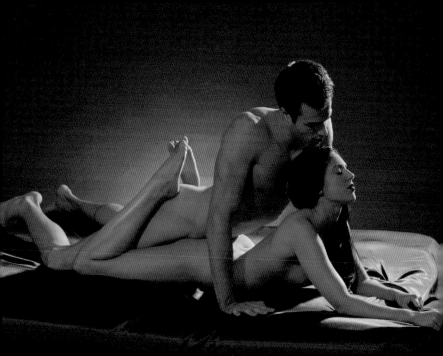

52 INSIDE OUT

With his legs tucked between hers, he has
little range of motion, which means she'll
be treated to quick in-and-out moves that'll
send waves of sensation to the nerve-packed
first few inches of her pleasure zone.

TWO-TIMING 53

Using his fingers and his tongue on
her at the same time is an easy way
to expand his repertoire while working
her into a heart-palpitating frenzy.

54 AMAZING ARC

She works hard in this pose, but she also reaps the booty bonuses. The curve of her body will put maximum pressure on her groin, while the rush of being upside down will send her overboard in no time.

THE EMBRACE 55

The pleasure of this pose lies in its close, loving contact, making it perfect for anyone who is truly intimate and only wants to get more so.

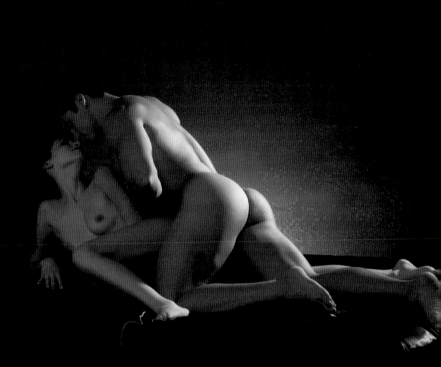

56 TEASPOONS

This very compact version of spooning is ideal for shallow penetration and targeted stimulation on the outer rim of the sex organs, where the nerve endings — on both him and her — are tightly packed.

TAKEOUT 57

This is the position of choice for public
encounters where time is a critical risk factor,
since the action can be shifted into fast-forward
by giving their orgasms a helping hand.

58 BODY BOOSTER

This pose raises rear entry to new heights as he enjoys the tight fit, but the slight lift on his groin adds just enough slow-down pressure to turn a fast-and-furious move into a more deliberate delight.

SLEEPING BEAUTY 59

She is sure to whisper, "My sweet prince has come!" when he slides into her from behind. She should twist so that her face isn't the only part of her waiting for his happily-ever-after kisses.

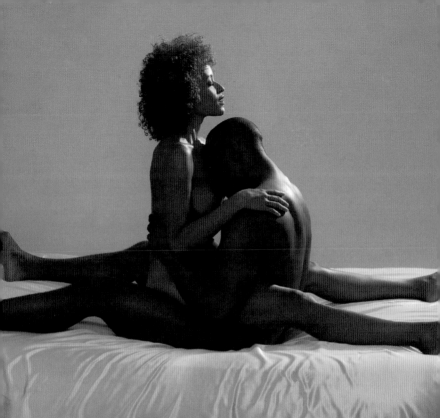

60 WINDMILL

When she sits in his lap with her legs spread, he will fit into her more directly, providing a deeper, fuller, more delightful feel. A little up-close-and-personal chest action doesn't hurt either.

TETHERBALL 61

This wanton, whimsical pose will up the erotic
ante for both partners. They can push and
pull with their arms and legs to tantalizingly
tease each other's whirling passion plays.

62 THE BUMP-AND-GRIND

She doesn't need to be a pro to give him a slow-burning lap dance — just strong thigh muscles to lower herself down on him in drive-him-wild circular motions. Va va voom!

BOOTY-GRAB 69 **63**

Hold the phone — this pose is certain to push
her buttons, since being on top means that she
gets to be in control at one end and feel his
strong hands on her backside at the other.

64 DOUBLE HEAD RUSH

Not a position for couples to do all night,
but then again, they won't need to. The
instant blood rush triggered when they
both lean face-down packs a powerful
intensity, heightening each thrust.

OTTOMAN EMPEROR 65

Placing his harem girl on a pedestal
puts her at his every command since her
precarious balancing act is at the mercy
of his powerful position behind her.

66 SITTING PRETTY

Besides the thrill of her gravity-defying acrobatics, he will also get pleasantly knock-kneed over being able to watch himself slide in and out of her.

GIRL ON TOP 67

She loves being on top because she gets to decide how hard and fast the action is; he loves it when she climbs up there because he gets to just sit back, relax and enjoy the sultry show.

68 GOOD VIBRATIONS

Get a buzz on. With the help of sex toys, it's a cinch to send her into orgasmic pleasure. Lying back is the perfect pose for her to give his magic wand full access to perform some XXX tricks and treats.

CIRCLE OF LOVE **69**

As he stays still, she can try rolling her
hips in a clockwise motion, then switch
to counterclockwise, then back again
every few seconds. The extra whirl will
add a racy spin to their romp.

He doesn't do much except provide the inside entertainment in this pose and then lie back and enjoy the show.

THE RIG 71

Drill, baby, drill. They'll both be gushing with joy in this intensely penetrating pose. When she holds on with a tight grip, she can control the pumping action for just the right rhythm.

72 OVERTIME

This move offers lots of room for extras — she can lean back a little bit to get greater G-spot stimulation, while he can use his hands to play dot-dot-dot with her love button and his mouth to tickle her toes.

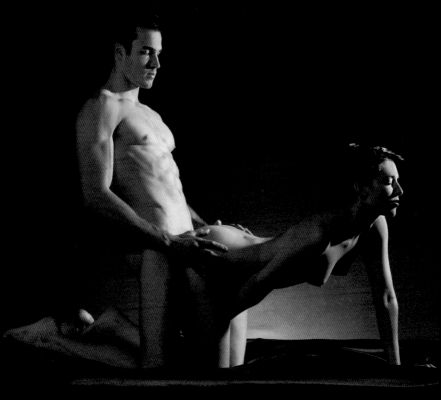

SNEAKY GIRL 73

It's easy for her to reach down between
her tight thighs and add to her personal
pleasure with a little on-her-own action.

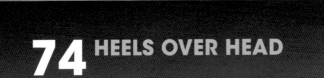

74 HEELS OVER HEAD

To get plenty out of this pose he needs to do just two things: lie back and feel the joy. However, he can also pull his legs down to encourage her to go lower and lower.

THE FIRM 75

Leaning back against a stable surface
will prevent any unwanted rolling from
stoppin' the action no matter how much
hoppin' and boppin' she does atop him.

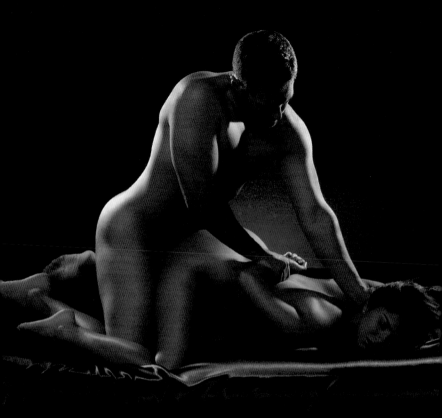

76 WRESTLING MANIA

He won't have to twist her arm to indulge
in a little rough-sex role-play — the erotic
incognito element of rear entry lends
itself perfectly to acting out carnally.

CAT 77

By sliding his hips a couple of inches higher up her body and rocking back and forth, he transforms standard man-on-top into the Coital Alignment Technique, which will positively make her purr with contentment.

78 CURLS

For those days when he wants to work his guns instead of burning his core, he can sit back and maximize the sensations by curling her up and down and gyrating her hips in a circular motion.

THREE-LEGGED RACE 79

The leg up in this position has two knee-trembling advantages: it makes for easy thrusting, and either partner can slide their hand down and make some finger magic.

80 SLIP-SLIDING AWAY

He can extend and expand his mounting move by lubricating her front side and then rubbing his whole body up and down in a slippery massage that will have her begging for the final slide inside.

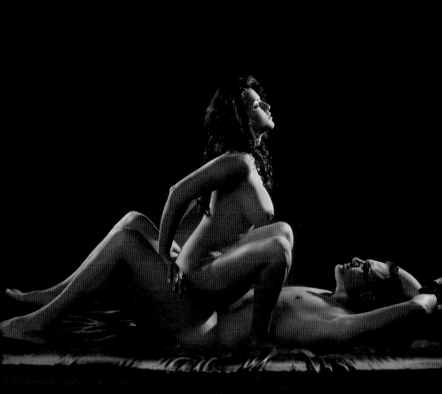

FIT TO BE TIED 81

She can make him her own private passion
plaything when she binds his hands and
climbs on top for a pleasure ride.

82 THE ANGLER

A dangling leg swung back and forth becomes orgasm bait — the wider she can cast it out, the bigger the climactic catch.

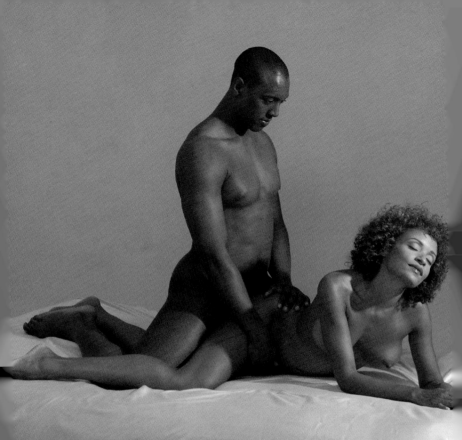

ARC DE TRIOMPHE 83

Because of the twisty positioning, the pleasure payoff will be all hers. By pushing up and arching her back as much as possible, she'll tighten things down below and give his hand an opening to march through.

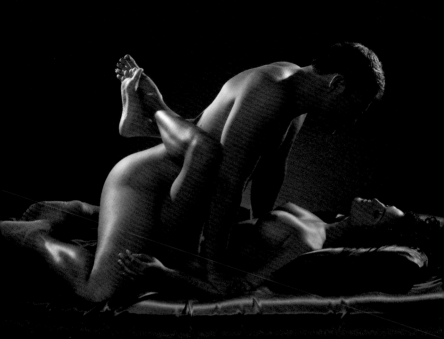

84 JELLYFISH

She can add to his joy by pulsing her legs ever so slightly. The added thigh movement will give him an extra rush in this already-tight fit.

CROSSED SPOONS 85

The old in-and-out won't work when partners snuggle up spoon-style, but crossing the two will get the job done. For him to stay inside of her, he will need to scoot his hips up and pulsate instead of stroke.

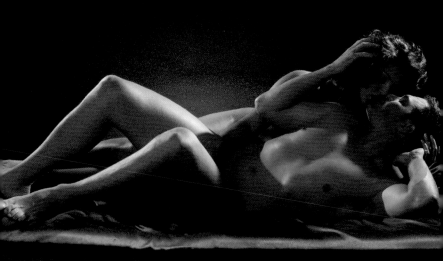

86 REVERSE SPOON

Here is her opportunity to bring him to
ecstasy by pleasuring him in a flesh-
to-flesh love-in that leaves room for
kissing, caressing and conversation.

LIFT AND SERVE 87

Standing sex has never been so easy.
She doesn't even have to lift her leg
high to make their stars align.

88 HOLDOVER

Tossing one leg over his shoulder is a
great way to improve access and an even
better way for her to keep her balance
if he makes her weak in the knees.

LEG LIFT 89

When his personal trainer is willing to sleep
with him to get the job done, working out
becomes a whole lot sexier! This position
will test his muscles as he holds his leg high
enough for her to work his equipment.

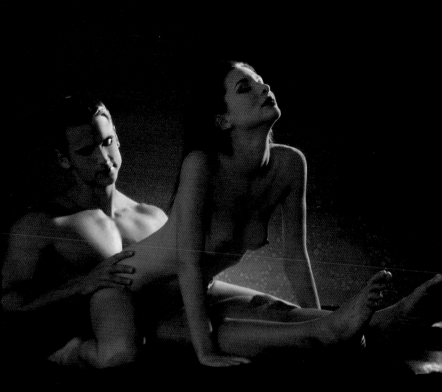

90 BACK UP

The fresh entry angle affords him a killer view of her pivoting posterior, giving him the opportunity to create all sorts of sweet new sensations. Hopefully he's a go-getter and will take the chance.

MARATHON **91**

To keep him deep down inside of her, she should wrap her legs tightly around his hips and squeeze hard with her pelvic-floor muscles. Her ecstasy grip will add some powerfully intense friction to his thrusts.

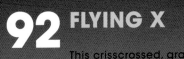

92 FLYING X

This crisscrossed, gravity-defying party trick will give both partners' orgasms a spine-tingling liftoff if they can master the high-wire act.

POGO 93

Having her feet on the bed allows her to pop up and down while he helps support her weight and holds her close to him and balanced upright above his stick.

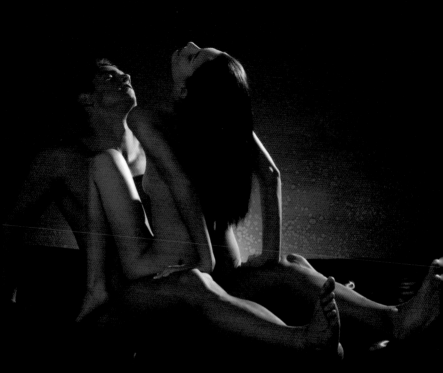

94 BUCKIN' BRONCO

This pose offers lots of leverage for red-hot riding. This means that both pardners can keep up a fairly steady rhythm without losing momentum as they gallop toward a real orgasmic round-up. Yeehaw!

GOLD STANDARD 95

There's a reason this is a best-of-the-best oral-sex pose for him — it puts her in a comfortable position with full access, it allows her to adjust up and down to any angle and it lets him simply lie back and enjoy.

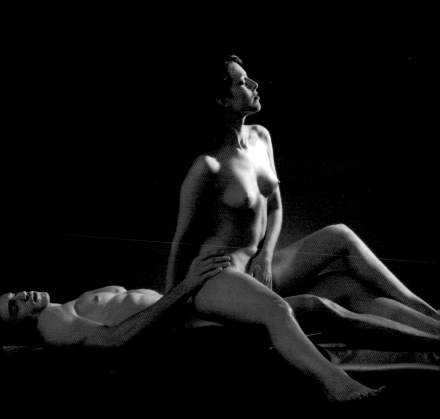

96 TWIN PEAKS

Stroking herself while doing the bump-and-grind gives twice as much titillation, which can launch her to an otherworldly orgasm.

FULL THROTTLE 97

She's in charge here, deciding how fast she wants him to go — and come. He's simply putty in her hands.

98 PIRATE'S BOOTY

She'll be happy that she walked his plank once his peg leg gets to work on her. The slight angular dip of his pelvis will make her feel like he is completely filling up her treasure chest.

VICE GRIPS **99**

With his arms outside her legs, she can communicate an astonishing amount of information about her pleasure with a squeeze here, a push here, and a final uncontrollable, suffocating constriction.

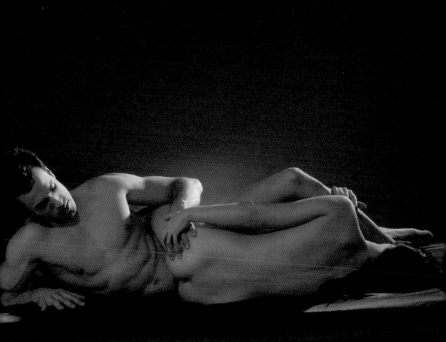

100 TWISTED EIGHTS

To double up the orgasmic delight, both partners should use ever-widening figure-eight motions so that he goes deeper and deeper in, rubbing up against her in long, sensuous strokes.

FETCH **101**

No doggy has ever enjoyed playing with a ball more. Instead of being buried in a mattress or getting burned on the carpet, her knees get to sit on the soft, bouncy ball and, well, bounce!

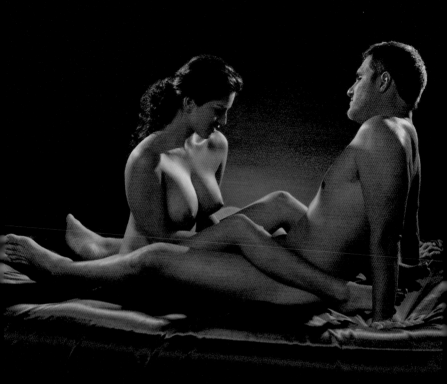

102 THE TEASE

This intimate position is ideal for deep eye contact and passionate kissing breaks as she builds and builds and builds his excitement.

TRAMPOLINE 103

This is a high-energy pose for the strong of heart (and arm for him) only. She should take care not to vault onto his groin with too much vigor, or she may end up breaking his bounce permanently.

104 CROSS OVER

Having him in a love grip with her thighs lets
her control the in-and-out and leaves him
free to use his hands to tickle, tantalize and
torment her (in the most wonderful ways).

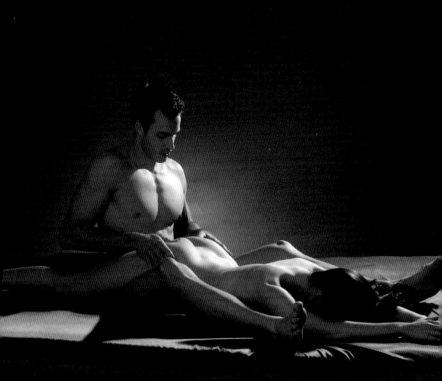

NAUGHTY RUMP **105**

He gets the double-bliss whammy of the curve of
her rear with an ultra-deep penetration, so even
though the movement is limited, he won't miss it.

106 BOYS ON THE SIDE

He'll be floored by this pose because it has all the relaxed ambience of going side to side, while she'll be sent flying by its woman-on-top flavor, which puts her completely in control of the action.

OUT OF SIGHT 107

He just can't beat the vista when she's lying
on her back. Her pose means that he can
watch her taking care of (his) business
and enjoy her curves at the same time.

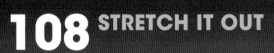

108 STRETCH IT OUT

A deceptively active move, it takes strong arms for her to set the pace so he can use his hips to help with some of the heavy lifting.

SUN SALUTATION 109

Flex time is sex time. Enlightenment is great, but mixing some yoga stretches into their lovemaking is going to have more of an immediate, extremely erotic benefit for couples: earthly bliss. Deep breathing necessary.

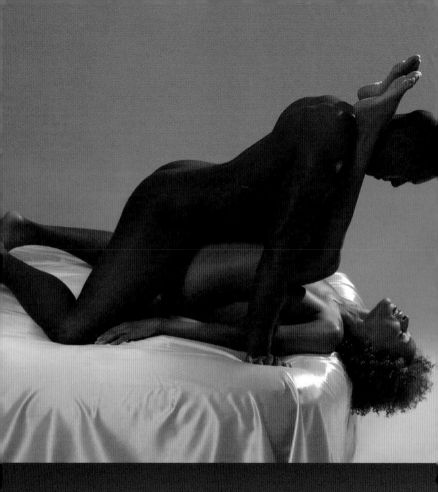

110 ON THE EDGE

The more forward he pushes her body, the farther upside down she will find herself and the closer she'll be to the edge of ecstasy.

THE ANCHOR 111

One of the more creative positions, this pose
can actually translate into hours of high-
friction fun once they get the balance right.
However, it takes plenty of arm strength
to really reap the risqué rewards.

112 THE VIRGIN

Crossing her legs to one shoulder as he thrusts will create that oh-so-tight feeling from the first time she ever had sex.

TOUCH AND GO **113**

When she sits on the side, it means all he has to do is reach in and let his fingers do the walking, dialing up her numbers to immeasurable heights.

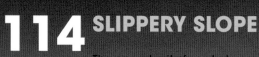

114 SLIPPERY SLOPE

The opportunity for a help-yourself orgasm is what transforms this from a run-of-the-mill ride to an extremely erotic rear-end romp.

WHO'S YOUR DADDY? 115

Spreading wide is going to give him a vulnerable feeling that she should freely exploit by aggressively getting what she wants. A few added slaps to the back of his thighs should remind him who's who.

116 THE RAMP

She may look like she's just lying there and enjoying the trip, but utilizing the area off the end of the bed to move her feet up and down allows her to easily control the angle and depth of his landing.

THE SLIDE 117

This is a tricky angle to master but it's worth it: the blood rush from her thighs is a heady aphrodisiac. She should make sure her neck is supported on his feet to avoid embarrassing-to-explain injuries.

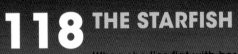

118 THE STARFISH

When she lies flat with her legs spread wide, he can press in as deep as both partners desire without worrying about uncomfortable pokes to her cervix.

TAKEOFF 119

Planting his feet wide will give her the
access she needs while creating a solid
base so that the bouncing fun doesn't
launch her in this oh-so-flighty pose.

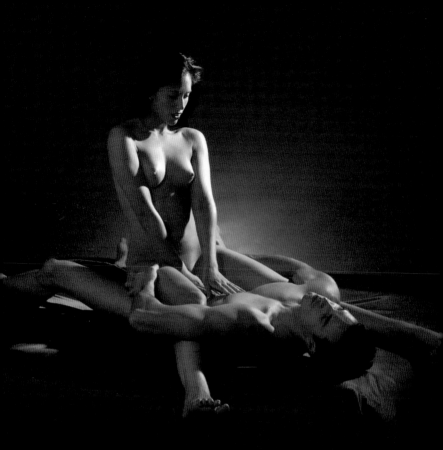

120 THE PLIÉ

Spreading her legs wide apart lets her control the action so that he can dabble for a bit at the edge of her pleasure dome instead of going in deep right away.

DOGGY REDUX 121

In this slight variation on the classic hound pose, she lies flatter, which changes the angle just enough for him to nudge against her G-spot with his bone.

122 ON A DEADLINE

This is a handy pose for a quick passion grope during those late nights at work. If she is wearing a skirt and he does a quick unzip, then this quick hop-on-hop-off position can be performed almost fully clothed.

HIGHWAY TO HEAVEN 123

She'll need strong legs and flexible knees for this one, but when she takes over the thrust-and-grind, it leaves him completely free to focus his attention on the rest of her body.

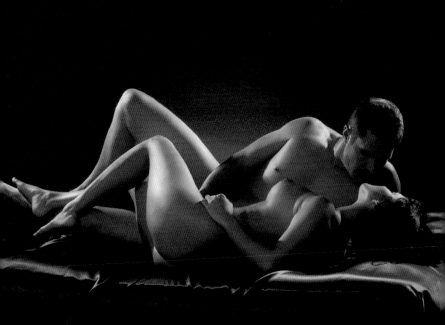

124 HOLD THE PICKLE

The relaxed tone of this pose combined with its sideways angle takes the pressure off of him and his parts, making it a favorite for guys who are quick on the draw.

STARTING BLOCKS 125

By bending one leg forward, she gains
a greater range of motion — including
circular — while her straight back leg will
produce added snugness that will have
them sprinting toward the finish line.

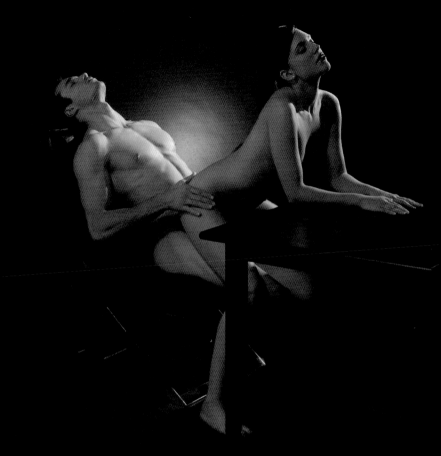

126 DESK SET

Leaning in opposite directions transforms chair sex from common to carnal in a configuration that is sure to rub them both the right way.

THE "Z" 127

The closer he brings his knees to his chest,
the easier it will be for her to pay some
amorous attention to his main accessory.

128 HEAD RUSH

This pose will give her a head-to-toe burst of pleasure as it increases blood flow to her head and changes her breathing pattern, mounting the feelings of sexual tension and arousal that a gold-medal orgasm thrives on.

TIGHTEN THE SCREWS 129

It may look like a trust-building exercise, but
when she clamps down tightly around him with
her pelvic-floor muscles, it is guaranteed to
bring their tryst to a sweet, speedy conclusion.

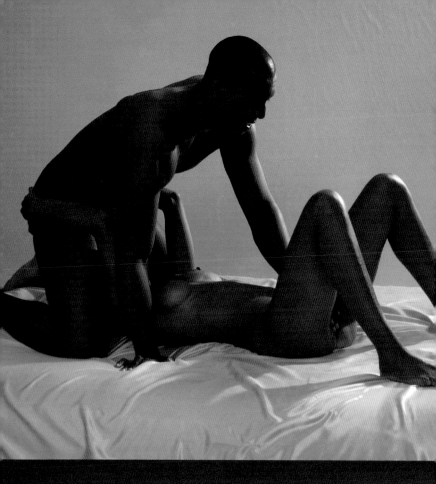

130 DOUBLE DARE

This pose makes it easy for him to manhandle her, but his bad-boy behavior may just break her concentration on him!

REAR END 131

This passion pose is unusual in that it is deeply relaxing for her while still giving him a pleasurable panorama of her posterior.

132 SPORTS FAN

If she has the stamina to pull this off, this position creates an incredibly snug fit, and the clear view means he can watch the game at the same time. He just needs to make sure that she also scores.

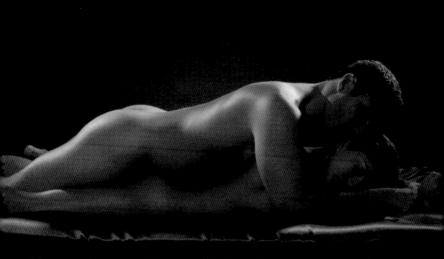

BELLY FLOP 133

This relaxing pose is incredibly comfortable for both partners without losing any of the pleasure — the angle is nearly perfect for him to go in deep and scorch her inner hot spots.

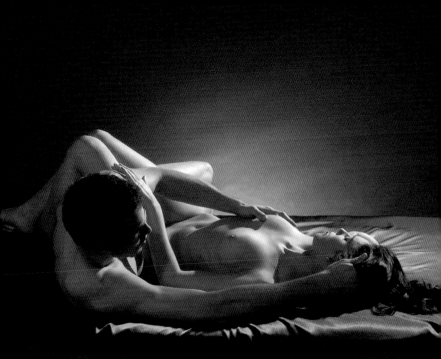

134 SKIN FLICK

Side-by-side positions give both partners
plenty of scope to massage and stroke
each other — the total skin-on-skin
contact is sumptuously steamy enough
to put them both in a moan zone.

THE CHIN REST 135

If she props her chin on her fist, with her
pinkie pointing down, she can use a finger
to put pressure on his perineum (the magic
bit of flesh between his balls and bottom).
Be ready, since he's likely to hit the roof.

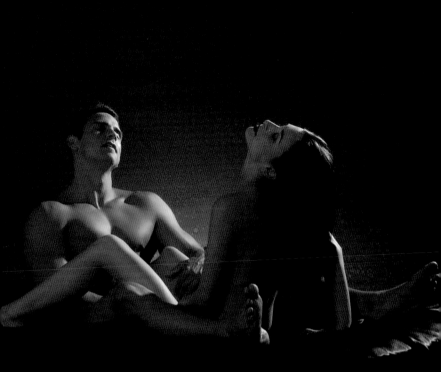

136 TANTRIC CUDDLE

This is a sweet, slow love lock with lots of
maneuver room for head-to-toe massages
and out-of-this world orgasms.

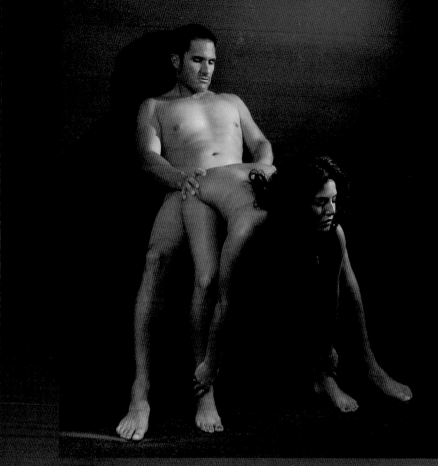

ON A TILT **137**

The fun begins when he leans back,
crushing their groins together in a hot,
juicy mash. She needs to push back so
they don't roll away from the wall while
he controls the up-and-down bounce.

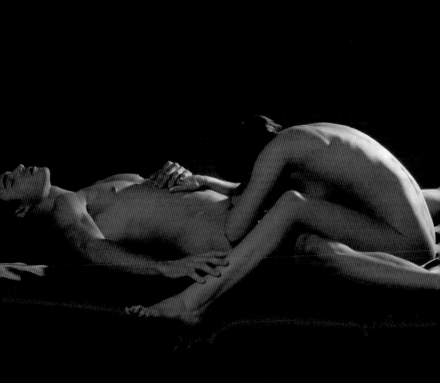

138 TWO-4-ONE

This is a great pose for her to take him
to the edge and then surprise him by
hopping on for a woman-on-top finale
before he knows what's hit him.

PRIME TIME 139

This young and restless pose has both partners positioned face-forward in their most comfortable TV-watching chair with a clear view of whatever action is on the screen.

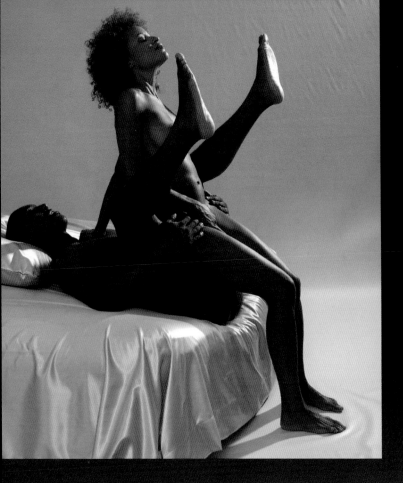

140 THE REV-IT-UP RUB

This woman-on-top/rear-entry combo gives
her a better shot at ecstasy because she
can easily pump her own O. He won't
mind — in fact, many guys get fired up about
a woman who knows how to self-service.

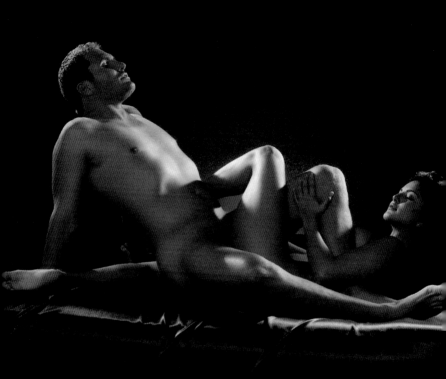

SPORK **141**

Lovers shouldn't worry about thrusting in
and out with this pose. The pleasure is
all in the pelvic muscles. A big flex isn't
necessary to feel the burn — small pulsating
squeezes should do the erotic trick.

142 THE BUTTERFLY

It doesn't take much to make the nectar-sweet sensations soar in this pose — both partners simply lie back and flutter their hips. The faster they wing it, the more intense the bliss.

HIDEAWAY **143**

Being on top can make her feel on stage and oh-so-overexposed. Cuddling up close and holding his hands will give her all the fabulous feelings of riding him without worrying that she is under the spotlight.

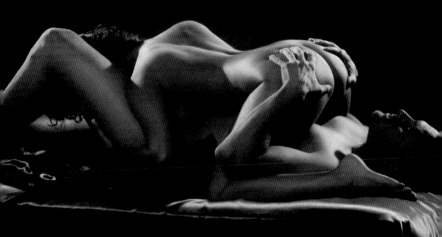

144 MUTUAL OF O

This tit-for-tat pose ensures that he can reciprocate the pleasure and lick rings around her rosie.

THE SURPRISE 145

It's this pose's very sweet simplicity that makes it the only move they'll need under their belt for when they want to slip away mid-party for a frisky frolic in a quiet corner.

146 SWORD SWALLOWER

She better be an expert to do this ultimate
deep-throat position. He is in control of the
thrusting, and the farther her head is over
the edge of bed, the wider her throat opens
to accommodate him without gagging.

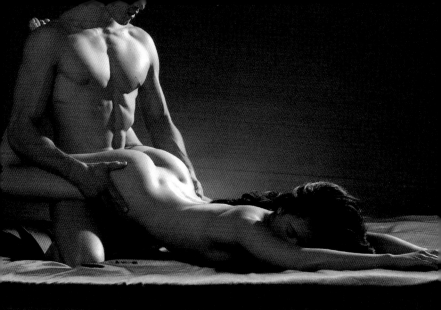

THE CRAWL 147

It looks relaxing, but this is actually a fairly vigorous position that gives both lovers the opportunity to thrust hard against one another to experience the deepest penetration possible.

148 THE WOW WOW

For this bottom-to-bottom bump to work,
he is going to need thighs of steel or
else give in to the impulse and simply
sit on her, which should make for some
very deep, meaningful sex indeed.

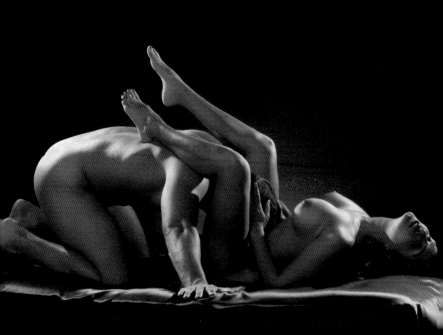

THE TUMBLER 149

By channeling her inner acrobat and
arching her back, she gives him full range
of motion to her entire love mat.

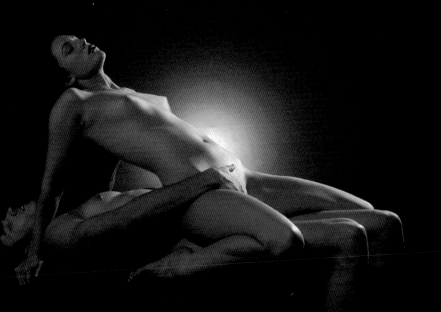

150 THREE-FINGER THRILL

A little firm, well-placed stroking can turn her cross-eyed with pleasure. He'll have to move fast to keep up with her racy routine.

THE MIXER 151

He can heat her up to red hot by gently rotating her legs back and forth, up and down, and all around as if he's stirring her. The move doesn't have to be anything big — a subtle spiral effect will be electric for her.

152 YAWNING POSITION

Tiny shifts in how each person balances their weight will change the direction of his dangle, bringing both partners to dizzying heights of pleasure. There is nothing boring about that!

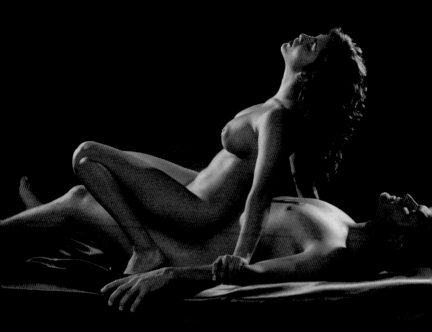

THE STALLION 153

If he has strong thighs, he can do all
the lusty labor by clenching his pelvis
rhythmically, gradually building up the
intense sensations while she holds on
tight and enjoys the torrid trot.

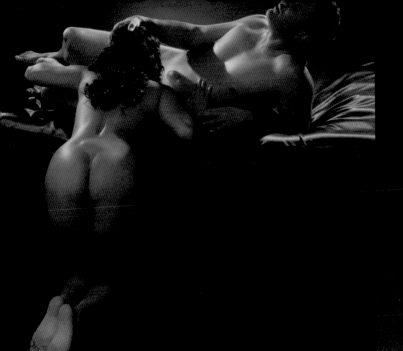

154 SIDEWINDER

Lying on his side adds an extra sensational slant to events as it lets her work the angle and slip in some extra handiwork.

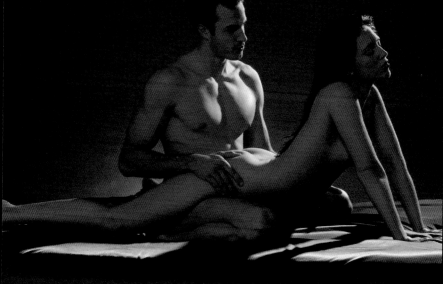

SEATED WHEELBARROW 155

There isn't enough leverage for him to do much in the way of raunchy rubbing in this pose, so all of the amorous action needs to come from her clenching her posterior and PC muscles in tiny passion pulses.

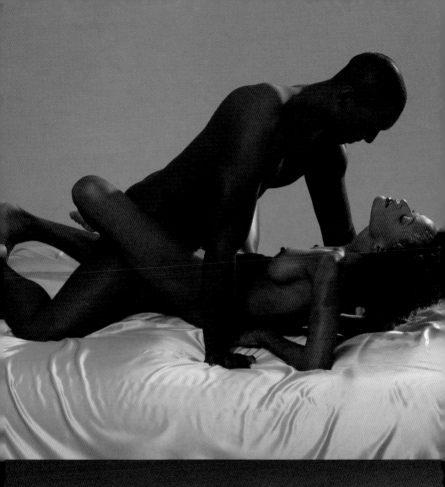

156 THE HOOK

This clasping position is fabulous for inducing the sort of muscular contractions that can move mountains.

STAND AND CARRY 157

She loves it when he carries her away, but not every he-man can sweep his partner off her feet. One trick is for him to lift her off of a table, holding her up by her feet instead of her legs.

158 THE CAMEL

This position may look a bit awkward, but if she's fairly limber and strong enough to hold her own weight, his hands will be free to give her babelicious curves the added loving attention they deserve.

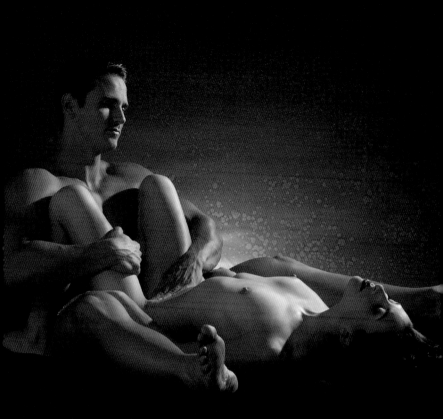

HOT SPOT 159

A wonderful way to ensure her blastoff is this
position, which produces no friction inside but
plenty of heat where she will enjoy it most.

160 TANTALIZING TEE-OFF

If she keeps her legs tightly together, he'll love the extra rub while she'll be able to feel every satisfying inch of him as he slides in and out of her.

BABE IN TOYLAND 161

Men hope that size doesn't matter; women are not so sure. But it's definitely true for vibrators — big or small, any energizer is fantastic for stimulating her all over and over the top.

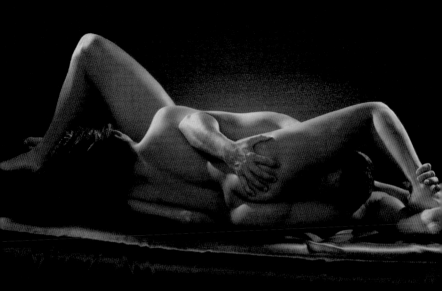

162 LAZY 69

Side-to-side oral is the perfect pose in case either partner wants to stop and take a quick breather midaction.

THE TIPSTER 163

When she slides a few pillows under her head, she stops him from dipping in too deep without cutting back on any of his oh-baby-yeah pleasure.

164 THE CARNAL CLENCH

Though this move offers megasensation, there isn't a lot of motion, so it's a prime pose for guys hoping to hold off on climaxing or couples who want to relish the feel of each other's bodies.

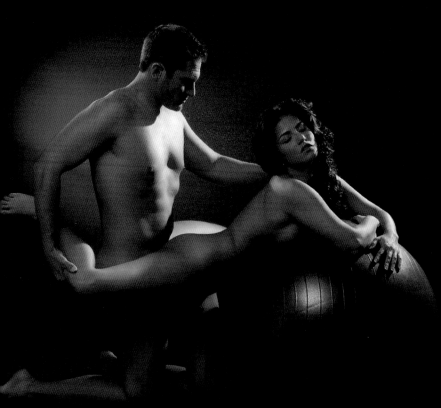

HEISMAN 165

Bringing a ball in on the action makes for award-winning nooky — she can tease him with fast up-and-down-the-field action, then cut back and go for wide, circular motions.

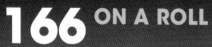

166 ON A ROLL

This superadvanced position uses an exercise ball to smooth out the usually bumpy ride that comes with her being on top, but slow, controlled up-and-down movements are best or she risks falling off.

THE SEXY BALLERINA **167**

Raising her leg like this will make it easier for him to give her his barre. It also slants her groin so that she gets some scorching sensual support exactly where she needs it while he practices his glissades.

168 SHIMMY SHIMMY SHAKE

He'll need iron willpower to make sure he does all the moving while keeping her perfectly balanced atop the ball. Even one tiny push forward on her hips will send her sprawling.

THE KNEELER 169

She loves this position because she gets
to balance herself over him just the
way she likes, but he should be warned
that she may practically suffocate him
when she hits her moan zone.

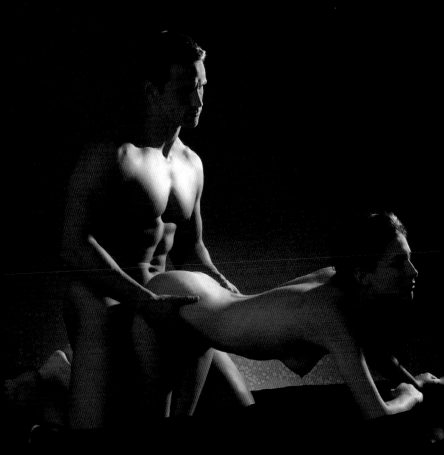

170 BLIND SPOT

One blissful bonus of this from-behind
position for her: Not being able to see
him lets her fully focus on all of the tingly
sensations going on behind the scenes.

THE CHEERLEADER 171

Give her an O! Give her an O! Gooooooo
O! He'll need to work fast to bring this move
to its climax, so he may want to warm
her up with a fingertip pep rally first.

172 CHAIR TRYST

It helps to hold on tight in this pose, but at least she won't have to worry about falling on the floor if he makes her knees buckle.

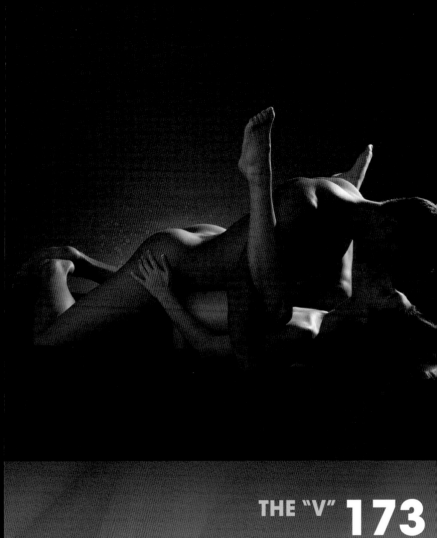

THE "V" 173

V is for victory in this deeply penetrating
and satisfying move. Hip-hip-hoorowza!

174 THE SCORPION

She can add a sweet sting to this move
by pinch-hitting with his bottom while
he tries not to lose his balance.

ELECTRIFIED 175

To hit her high note even faster, she can
multitask — here, sitting in reverse cowgirl
stimulates her inner back wall, while
using an erotic electronic on herself adds
plenty of instant all-over excitement.

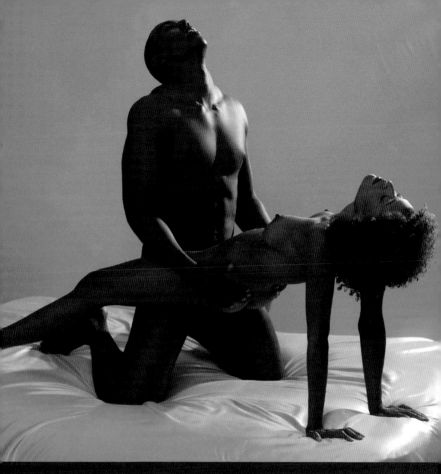

176 DRAWBRIDGE

This pose is not for the weak, but if they can hold it, they will both adore the completely centralized sensation of their groins merged and grinding away against each other.

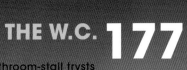

THE W.C. 177

Staying vertical is crucial to bathroom-stall trysts because it keeps naked flesh off of questionable surfaces and is fairly easy to do in tight spaces.

178 DRIVER'S SEAT

Ignore the speed limit! When she holds his head and opens her legs wide, she gets to choose where to steer him while deciding exactly how fast or slow she wants him to get there.

TAKE ME TO YOUR LEADER **179**

Even though she's on top, he's in charge. So
she gets to relax while he takes full control
to go as fast, slow, or deep as he pleases.

180 THE PRAYING MANTIS

The upward tilt of her pelvis means his tool
will be able pull double duty and rub her
inside and out. He'll need to hold on tight
because that sort of multitasking practically
guarantees her a no-hands multiple O.

POSSESSION 181

This is a very erotic and intimate position because they can extend the passion with lots of kissing and touching. The longer the buildup, the more powerful and exciting the climax when they finally let go.

182 LITTLE BIRDY

She'll feel like she's flying when she pushes off from his thighs with total abandon, and he'll feel extremely grounded because the harder she presses, the deeper into her he goes.

STEP UP 183

His raised leg will help support her weight so that their arms don't get tired before they reach the finish. A staircase is another ideal place to put this position into blissful action.

184 HOKEY POKEY

He puts his right hand in, he puts his right hand out, she puts both her hands in and she shakes 'em all about — that's what it's all about!

THE HIP LIFT 185

Once they have some serious momentum, she should surprise him by lifting her hips without warning so that he pops out. Then after hovering for a second she can move back down on him. Repeat as needed.

186 CHAIR LIFT

This scorching spin on rear entry is perfect for I-need-you-now quickies. The tension she feels in her torso from holding the pose means that she'll be on a big-bang fast track.

BACK DIVE 187

In this clever pose, she'll be able to revel in throw-the-head-back abandon while magically keeping them from thrusting off the end of the bed by locking her arms in place.

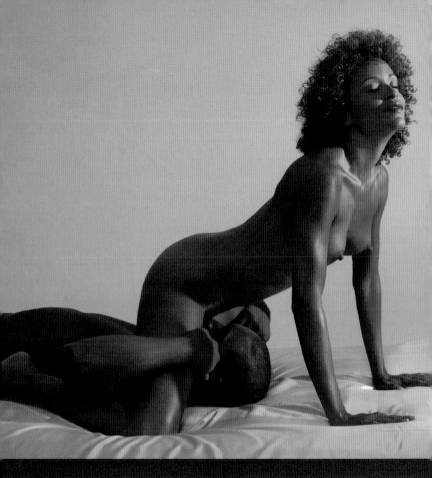

188 STRADDLE UP

The pleasure never stops — her bottom
and breasts are just a short reach away
from his groping hands with this pose.

FANTASY ISLAND 189

She can close her eyes and give in to the sweet sensation of being stroked as her imagination wanders — maybe it's that charming doctor or cute waiter or sexy VP from the Milan office or...

190 TABLE TOP

Woman-on-top comes in handy for some impromptu hors d'oeuvres whenever their carnal appetite needs satisfying, and standing on the chair wisely keeps her knees off the hard wooden table.

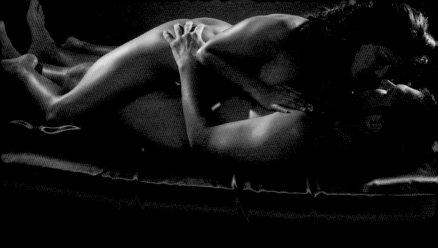

HER MISSIONARY 191

This flip on missionary is comfortable and intimate, which makes her feel seductive and sensual and all but guarantees an earth-shattering climax. But beware — she may never want to just lie on her back again.

192 COURTING CHAIRS

Varying the location from bed to chair — or, in this case, two chairs — can be enough to pump up the beat of that same old song into a hot new boogie.

WHEELBARROW 193

Both partners can add to the excitement with this pose. While he supports her body and controls the main movement, she should arch her back to better thrust her groin against him.

194 THE BODYGUARD

Holding his legs helps her keep a regular romp rhythm while working in some just-happened-to-be-in-the-neighborhood bottom caresses at the same time. Of course, he can also return the favor.

69 MASSAGE 195

With her on top in this 69 he can treat her booty to an erotic massage while keeping her legs wide enough to give him a great angle on her hot spot.

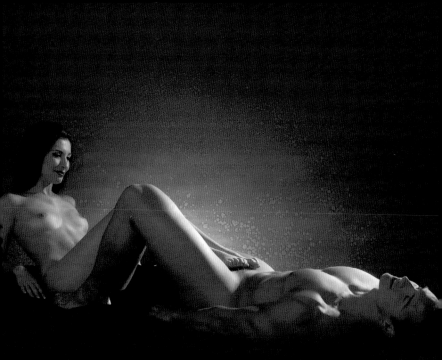

196 FOOTSIE

When she uses her feet to satisfy him,
she's also arousing herself for the return
favor. The foot-sensation area of the brain
is next door to the region that registers
the bliss-o-meter levels of the genitals.

WALK THE WALL 197

She may be lying down, but her stride will
be the primary force in this pose. She can
march her feet up and down his chest to
adjust the angle of penetration until she
finds the formula that works best for her.

198 RIDE 'EM, COWBOY

Lovers can create loads of feel-good friction in rear entry by propping up their upper bodies ever so slightly. He may just need to hold on once she starts bucking.

CARNAL CLUTCH 199

Rather than just moving up and down,
which can be tiring for her and leave
her less time to concentrate on her own
pleasure, she can try grinding forward and
back, rubbing her groin against his.

200 THE BUFFET

This tasty move lets him have a sample of all she has to offer. Plus she can peek down at his hot plate, unless opening her eyes combined with the blood rushing to her head makes her too dizzy with pleasure.

LONDON BRIDGE **201**

If she's apprehensive about being on top,
they can try this smooth maneuver: while
lying on the bed in a tight, canoodling
embrace, they simply roll together so
that — voila — she's riding his upper deck.

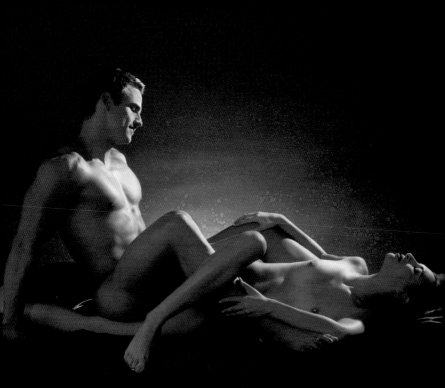

202 ROCK, PAPER, SCISSORS

Although it looks twisty to get into, this is actually a fairly relaxed pose, but one with little room for movement. The lusty sensations will result from short contractions of their inner thighs in unison.

RAUNCHY WRESTLER 203

This is not a hold than can be maintained
for long, so wait until the final round. They
will need to plant their legs firmly to get
enough lusty leverage for strong thrusting.

204 MIDAIR DOCK

Lying sideways at the end of the bed with
her legs spread into space really opens
her landing pad. He should work his hips
back and forth as well as side to side
to crash-land on her sexiest spots.

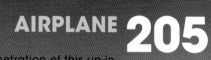

AIRPLANE 205

The deep, intense penetration of this up-in-
the-air pose will send her spinning into
the stratosphere, no air bag required.

206 REVERSE THE RIDE

The simplest positions are often also the best ones, losing nothing on the pleasure front just because they're easy to do. In this turned-around cowgirl configuration, all both partners need to do is close their eyes and feel the love.

SIT-IN 207

Each of them is firmly grounded in this pose, so it's the perfect opportunity to bend, reach, and twist to anywhere on the other's body and ignite that spot with light, fluttery, barely there kisses.

208 HEAVEN KNOWS

With their bodies totally bonded, they should go fast enough to get their hearts beating but slow enough that they will each feel the other's pounding away.

TWO-HEADED SNAKE 209

She'll think that his genitals have
sprouted an extra helpful organ when
he gets his hand in on the act.

210 LADIES' CHOICE

In this dual-purpose pose, he can slide in her front or rear end. It might take a bit of practice to get it right, but hey, who's complaining? She can wiggle around until it feels oh-so-right.

THE LUSTY LIE-IN 211

This low-energy carnal cuddle is perfect for those lazy days when one or both partners want some extra tawdry action that is outside of the bedroom, but without the athletic effort.

212 EASY RIDER

The easiest way for him to slide in and out when she's on top is for her to rest against the bed for support and lift her body up and forward so that she can push back down the bed opposite his thrusts.

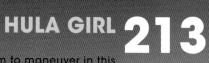

HULA GIRL **213**

He has plenty of room to maneuver in this
pose so she can gyrate her hips side to
side to create her private orgasm dance.

214 SINKHOLE

Sitting on his feet and wrapping her legs around him allows for some of the deepest penetration while also lifting and fully opening her for some added manual stimulation.

TWIZZLER 215

If he can rub his belly and pat his head at the same time, then he will be able to swivel her hips in tiny circles while he rocks back and forth, ensuring a mind-blowing climax for both of them.

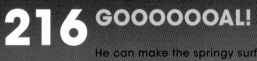

216 GOOOOOOAL!

He can make the springy surface work for him by thrusting his tailbone back when she bobs up. The rebound bounce makes a surprise impact on her love button.

SPIDER 217

When he's on top, he can push too hard. By keeping her legs bent, she can push up with her body to let him know when he's coming on too strong.

218 THE CUDDLER

This is a slow-building, easy-orgasm position,
which means there's plenty of time for
him to whisper sweet — or nasty — things
to her while nibbling her lobes.

SWEET SEAT 219

This unusual and challenging twist on the 69 pose is sure to ratchet up the passion for both partners, but she will only enjoy it if the chair has plenty of padding since there will be a lot of pressure on her shoulders.

220 THE CORKSCREW

The tight angle of this pose combined with the pressure of his groin means that all she has to do is rotate her hips to pop her cork.

AVALANCHE 221

To stop her from falling flat on her face, they will need to keep their below-the-belt regions extra meshed. If she feels herself slipping, she can use her legs to squeeze tight and keep the carnal connection.

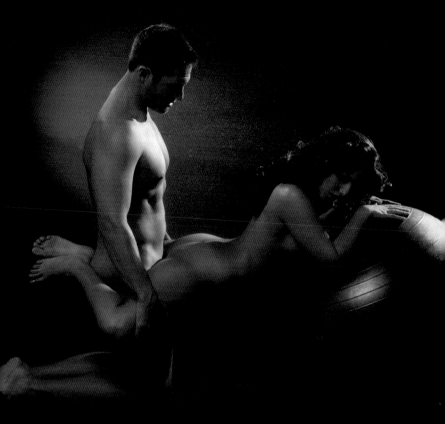

222 BIG WHEELBARROW

Pushing her back and forth as he plows her field will certainly reap a raunchy harvest.

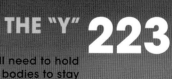

THE "Y" 223

For this move to work, they'll need to hold strong to each other's bodies to stay together. On the plus side for her, his hand has easy access to the action area.

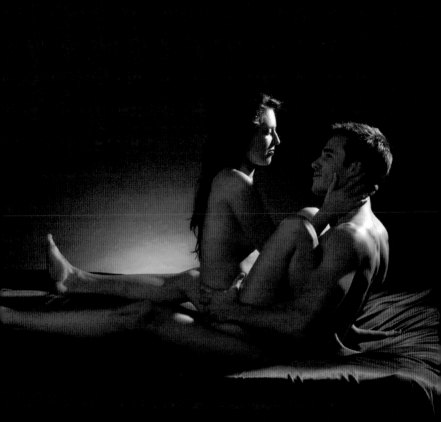

224 THE FLOWER BUD

This oh-so-intimate version of woman-on-top
works in some intense eye contact and brings
them close enough to caress and lock lips.

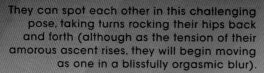

THE CLIMBER 225

They can spot each other in this challenging
pose, taking turns rocking their hips back
and forth (although as the tension of their
amorous ascent rises, they will begin moving
as one in a blissfully orgasmic blur).

226 DOWNWARD DOG

The downhill angle of this pose makes for a moan-inducing tight fit. He may need to do some deep breathing to hold off "ohming" too quickly.

COOL HAND LUKE **227**

He loves when she's on top and he can play with her breasts; but in this pose his hands stay busy creating heat by moving her body, so she gets to thrill them both by playing away with her hot little hands.

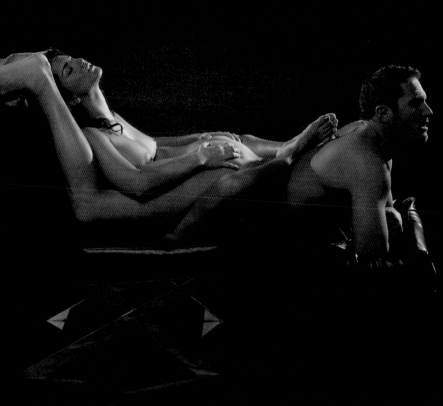

228 ROW, ROW, ROW

This is actually a fairly cozy pose that will rock both his and her boats, with tiny thrusts of both partners' hips propelling the action.

THE TIPPING POINT 229

Balancing acts are a great way to add an exciting edge to erotic play. The thrill of feeling the chair rock precariously with every thrust will send their adrenaline levels skyrocketing.

230 GET INTO THE GROOVE

She is well-balanced to play with different rhythms, so she can move her hips in a steady circular motion or jig back and forth to make him work like a probe seeking to reach all of her pleasure zones.

ALL HANDS ON DECK 231

He will turn her to putty with this two-handed massage trick. Gently pressing on the secret hot spot about three inches below her belly button helps boost blood flow for a yowza effect on the whole pelvic area.

232 FRONT AND REAR

The tricky angle is worth it when it means
that he can reach down or around and
twiddle her hot buttons, front and rear.

THE SWING 233

The sexy sweat, the revved-up rubbing, the frenzied friction, the plunging penetration, the passionate pressure, the racy rhythm — these are all key elements of sexual combustion.

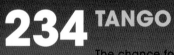

234 TANGO

The chance for overloading on skin contact makes this pose scorchingly sexy right away, but having the ball support her as she arches her body upward gives him the extra-smoldering view of her ecstasy.

REVERSE JOCKEY 235

One reason she should straddle up: When
he's on top, he has to support his weight
so he doesn't crush her, but when she's the
rider, he can relax and savor every sensation,
which makes him very, very grateful.

236 PASSION PRESS

When a couple is not within the same height range, the best way to get it together on the run is for her to kneel on something. Pushing her legs together will reap big climactic rewards for both partners.

DOING LAPS 237

Rather than working with the motion of his ocean, pushing down hard against him with her hips will give her the firm pressure she needs.

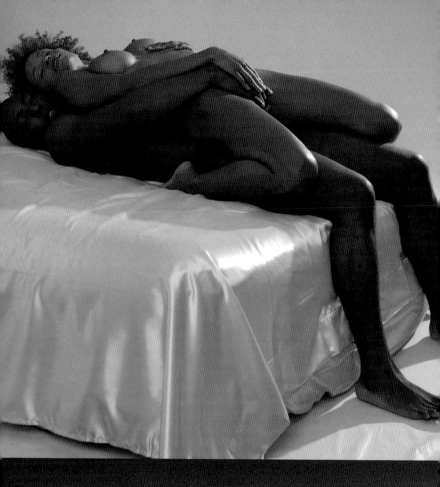

238 LUST LESSON

He will find it totally wanton when she acts like his tawdry tour guide, taking him downtown on a trip of exactly what kind of strokes make her vocal.

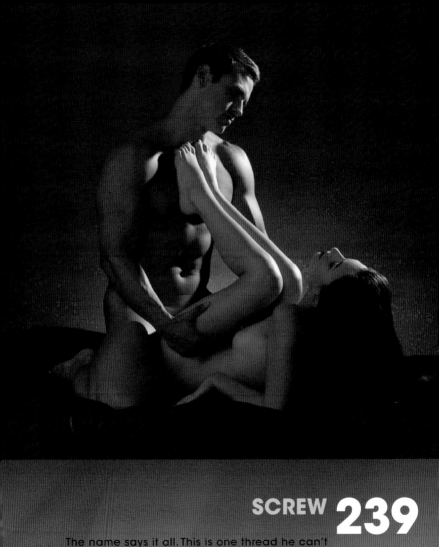

SCREW 239

The name says it all. This is one thread he can't
strip even if he gets overexcited, so he should
swirl her hips in small concentric circles, going
faster and faster until he hammers her home.

OVER THE EDGE

Dangling her leg in everwidening circles guarantees the sort of buzzy vibrations that will make them both want to come back for more and more.

THE DOWN LOW 241

Leaning her upper body forward as low as she can go has the double-whammy effect of pumping her G-spot while giving him a lewd look at her private parts thrusting against his.

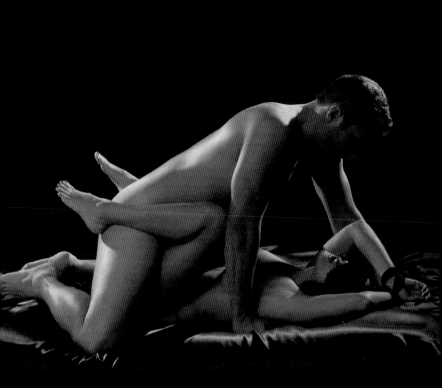

242 BLIND LOVE

Every caress and touch is that much more intense when she can't see what he is about to do. He can up her anticipation with surprise moves such as unexpected licks, kisses, and caresses.

BOOT IT UP 243

Usually rump romps are tightly bent affairs
with both partners in extreme embrace
to make the fit work, but in this pose, the
creatively arranged furniture frees their
movement for a very different experience.

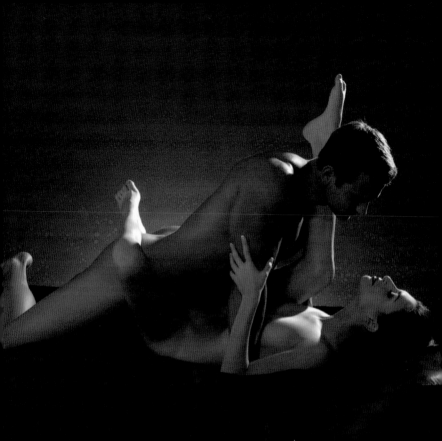

244 THE LIFT

All it takes to boost the basic missionary
out of the same-old, same-old is a simple
leg lift. The higher she inches up either leg
on his body, the steamier things will get.

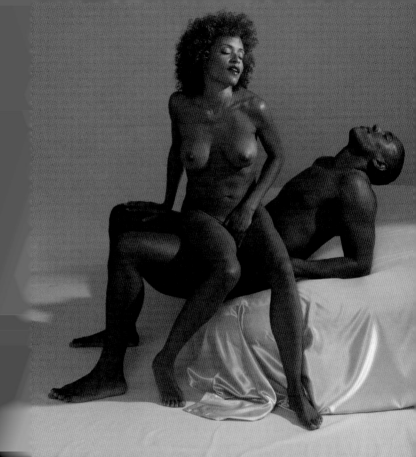

SIDE SLIDE 245

While this pose couldn't be hotter, it's not the easiest to put into action. He will need to have very strong legs to support her extracurricular activities, so she should work hard and fast at pleasing him as well as herself.

246 PICNIC TABLE

Enjoying some outdoor excitement doesn't need to be a dirty affair. This rear-entry pose creates a pleasingly snug fit, and they can get into it without even dropping their jeans below their knees.

LAUNCH PAD **247**

Lifting his legs high in the air puts him in a completely exposed pose that's perfect for hitting all the points on his rocket booster — his bottom, testicles, perineum, and shaft. She should be prepared for instant liftoff.

248 MUSICAL CHAIR

With her feet on the ground and his hands
pushing up on her bottom, this is the easiest
face-sitting position for starting and stopping.
She should sit, stand, sit, stand...until she
is teased to an orgasmic crescendo.

PUSH-UP 249

He'll need a lot of power in his arms to keep the thrusts turbocharged in this high-energy pitch on rear entry.

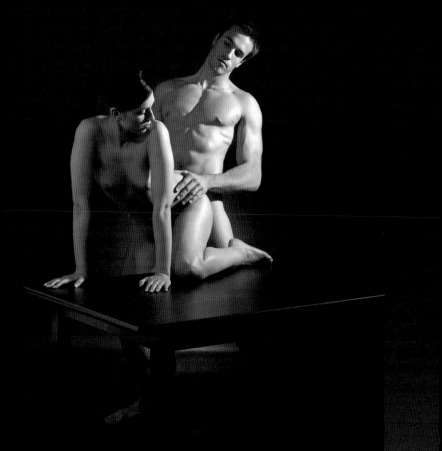

250 HANDRAIL

The key to making standing rear entry
work is all about matching heights — lifting
her leg high helps turn this tricky position
into a point-and-shoot moment that's
perfect for an on-the-go quickie.

HOT CROSS BUNS **251**

Rather than a straightforward in-and-out,
she should rock gently backward and
forward while he swivels his hips in small
circular motions to pump up the pleasure.

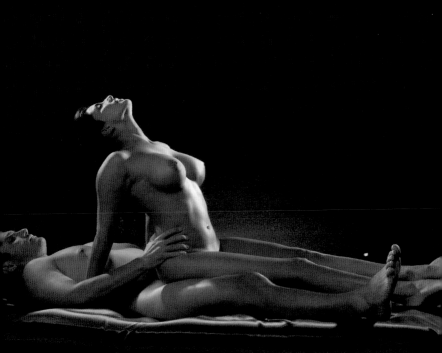

252 ON THE SPOT

The whole landscape changes when she turns her back to him, so although he has a hard time hitting all of her inner hot spots in most other positions, he will have a hard time missing them in this one.

HORNY HORSEY **253**

This position is all about megadeep penetration, so it's best to have a well-oiled saddle before he starts riding.

254 OFFICE PLAY

To earn his end-of-the-year bonus, he should keep her tilted forward and move her hips in a circular motion. If her legs aren't long enough to straddle him, she can gain a few extra inches by keeping her high heels on.

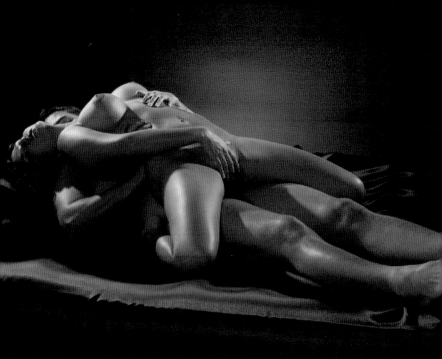

TRIPLE X **255**

For some X-rated action that adds a whole new level of lust, he can massage her breast and nibble her ear while she lends a helping hand to what is already a scorching pose. You go, girl!

256 HIGHER PLANE

She will feel like she is floating on a cloud
even before her orgasm — she can lie back,
breathe deep, and let him rock her to ecstasy.

THE PIN-UP 257

She'll give him a standing ovation when he
presses her up against the wall and pays
homage to what's between her legs.

258 THE DUMBBELL

Twisting her torso back and forth can turn their love session into a lusty workout, whittling her waist while pumping up his favorite muscle.

THE MAGIC SLIDE 259

It's all in the angle of the legs — the higher she raises them, the bumpier her ride. He can add a few moguls and tilt against her in all of the right places by rocking back and forth instead of pumping up and down.

260 LOVE BUG

With her completely hidden from his view, this position is his opportunity for a secret fantasy. As she provides the physical pleasure, he should let his imagination take flight for the ultimate mental stimulation.

BUTTERFLY IN FLIGHT 261

With her legs spread ceiling to floor and his back leg providing ample leverage, they are sure to experience plenty of fast-fluttering action in this position.

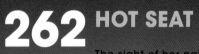

262 HOT SEAT

The sight of her naked on his lap and pumped up with passion is guaranteed to make him go ga-ga. She should go with the vixen vamping and exaggerate her movements while moaning loudly enough to wake the neighbors.

NUTCRACKER **263**

She should squeeze her thighs together to
press his groin into a stiff holding pattern
for a snug fit that will help keep the
balance — it will also make him seem bigger
and everything feel deliciously tighter.

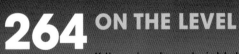

264 ON THE LEVEL

If there is a huge height difference, a footstool or stairs will even things out for standing sex without him having to support her weight (making it ideal if he — or she, for that matter — hasn't been to the gym recently).

THE ARCH 265

Holding herself slightly elevated gives him
a target worth shooting for. As he fires
away, she is free to slant her back so his
upward thrusts hit just the right spot.

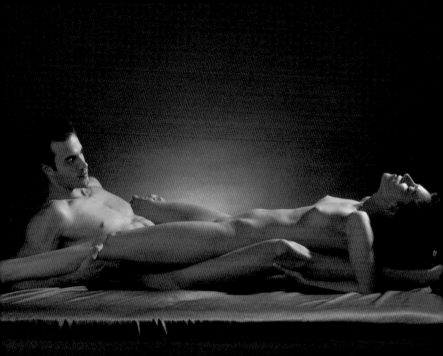

266 FULL EXPOSURE

Leaning back will show off her full-frontal assets to their best advantage by making her stomach look flatter and her breasts perkier.

SLOWLY DOES IT **267**

This kind of carnal connection isn't about insta-orgasm, it's about savoring every sensation. Partners can cuddle up in this pose and glide their hands over each other's bodies to uncover new pleasure points.

268 THE THRONE

In this royal position, the king and queen can share power by taking turns controlling the movement. She can rock for a while then stop and let him do some thrusting. It works great as long as only one partner rules at a time.

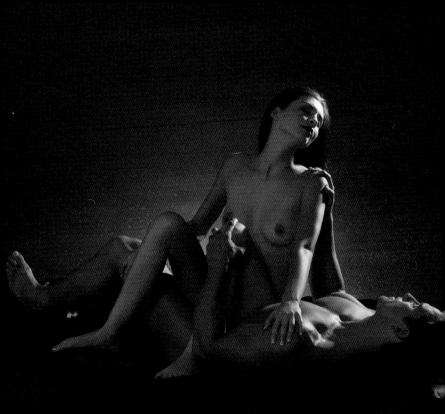

SCREW IT TIGHT **269**

This pose creates a really snug fit, making
it just the thing for when she craves a
supertight fit or when he's on the small
side (not that she'd ever tell him).

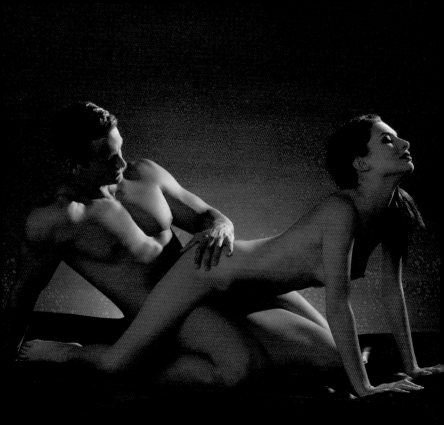

270 REVERSE COWGIRL

Even though she's the one who decides how
hard and fast they ride in this pose, he can
always give her a soft love tap if she slows
down to a trot when he's looking to gallop.

THE BALL BOB **271**

The tasty promise of a little lip-ercize on
a stability ball is sure to keep any couch
potato committed to their workout plan (she
may just want to slip in a few toe curls).

272 THE ULTIMATE HUG

With her arms and legs locked around him,
they can't get any more up-close and personal.
What is lost in free movement is more then
made up for in longing looks and deep kisses.

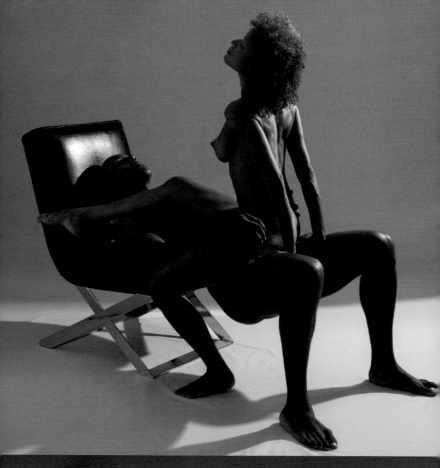

THE GO AROUND 273

She can swivel her leg over him to twist in an
around-the-world raunchy rotation that may
leave him never wanting to get up again.

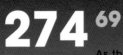

274 ⁶⁹

As the saying goes, it's better to give than it is to receive... but when it comes to sex, it is much, much better to give and receive at the same time!

THE SHOULDER HOLDER 275

Any time she raises her legs, it narrows her love canal and puts her in perfect position to control how he stimulates her G-spot. The "so-what" is that her orgasm will be peel-her-off-the-ceiling wonderful.

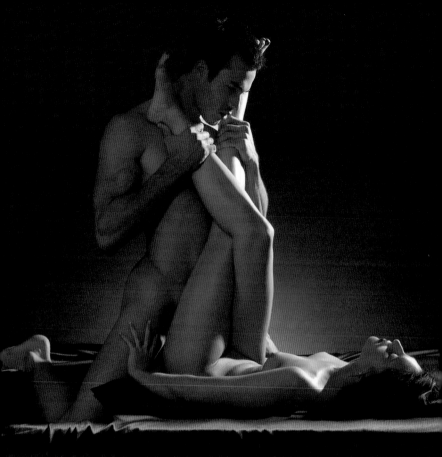

276 SCISSORS

He opens and closes her limbs with every thrust, stretching her from pleasingly wide open to totally titillating tight. From deep to squeezed, each stroke will give her something new to moan about.

MILE-HIGH CLUB 277

This is a sweet pose for making love in tight quarters like an airplane bathroom. They don't need much room since she tucks into his lap and lets his capable hands move her just right.

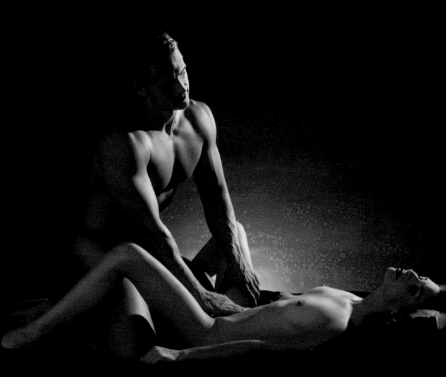

278 LADY IN WAITING

Not for a shy girl, this extremely wide-open position has her lie back and think of pleasure, luxuriating in the loving attention he is able and willing to give her.

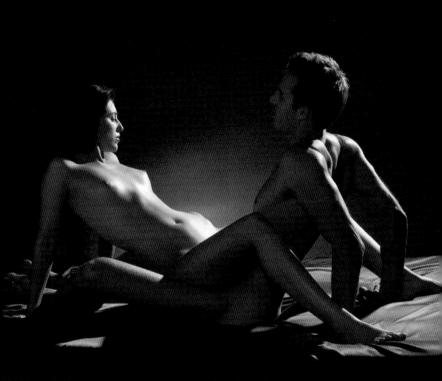

THE FUSION **279**

Because they are connected at the
groin, this pose calls for subtle squeezes
to keep their bodies merged as one.

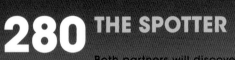

280 THE SPOTTER

Both partners will discover some new
O-zones when he lifts her leg and
adjusts the angle of penetration.

HOT-SPOT SUPERHERO 281

By opening herself up in this way, she can help
her superman tantalize all of her pleasure zones.

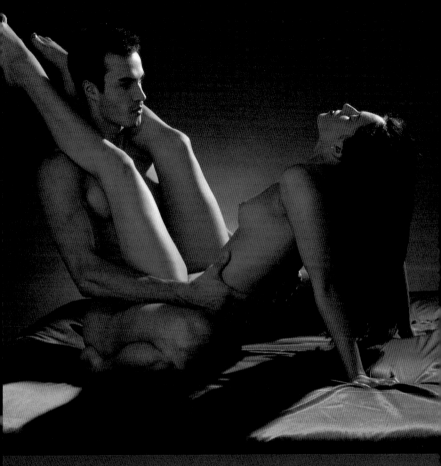

282 WATERSLIDE

He should hold her firm enough that he not only slides her back and forth on his spout but also helps support her weight so her arms don't collapse before splash down.

THE TENDER EMBRACE 283

As he pumps and enjoys the action shot,
he can look up at her face and take in all
the bliss he's bringing her. Then he'll want
to do it again...and again...and again....

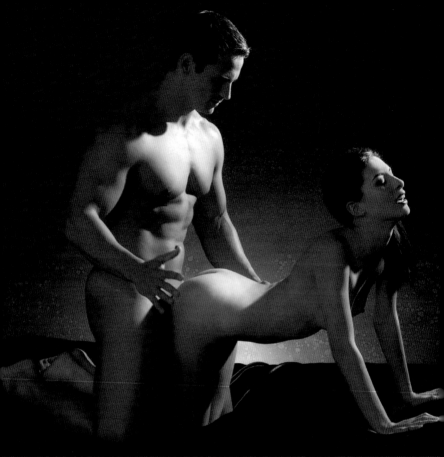

284 CANINE CANOODLING

Doggy position is an all-purpose move no matter
what size he is — the angle of the dangle means
there is never any danger of him slipping out,
no matter how hot and heavy the action gets.

UP-CLOSE AND HOT 285

This hybrid pose gives plenty of opportunity for soulful eye gazing while losing none of the raunchy rewards a good pelvis grind reaps.

286 NECKING

He should look for erogenous zones all over her body. His kissing, licking, and nibbling on her neck will greatly amplify the clitoral stimulation to give her an old-fashioned, drive-in movie petting session.

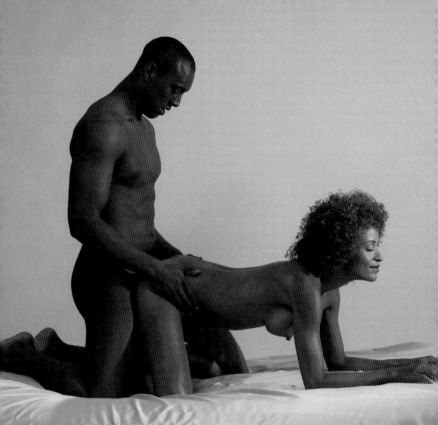

DEEP DIVE 287

Classic rear entry is a fairly tight pose, but if he wants to fish in even deeper waters, he can grasp her hips and pull her in toward him.

288 PLAY BALL!

With its soft seat and open access, an exercise ball can be a great sex chair. But watch out for the bounce! If they are not careful, his bat might go a few innings deeper than she expected.

BOTTOM JIG 289

Her booty is practically begging for his
touch in this primo posterior position.

290 LUSTY LAUNCH

The extra tension of pulling in opposite directions will add a thrilling tension to their thrusts. If they keep the hold until liftoff, it will add a turbocharged surge to their climax.

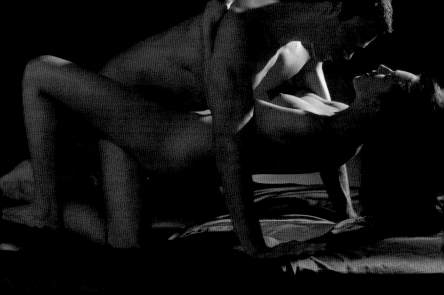

ELEVATED JACKHAMMER 291

The name says it all. With the old jackhammer,
he controlled the speed, depth, and force
of penetration. Now she meets him halfway
to double the power-tool pounding.

292 BELLY DANCER

This totally tingly pose gives both partners plenty to get excited about. He can easily stroke and caress her as she gyrates her hips in soft circular motions, literally seducing him with her body.

BEACH BONFIRE 293

When they don't want to get sand in intimate places, she can keep things clean by leaning over and holding her legs to brace herself. He needs to hold her tight as they hang ten, or she'll do a face-first wipeout.

294 WORLD'S STRONGEST

He'll need legs — and a will — of steel before
attempting this one or else he might drop
her as she makes him weak at the knees.

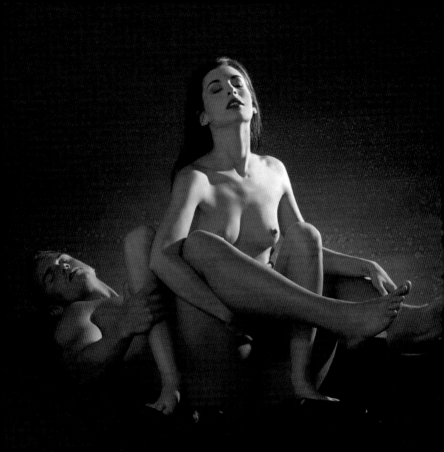

G-FORCE 295

This on-the-back maneuver guarantees a
direct hit on her G-spot, but his limited range
of motion means she will need to do the
pumping to avoid going into a free fall.

296 RISE AND SHINE

This one is so easy, they will want to do it again and again. The snug fit will create waves of pleasure for both of them. If she wants to change the sensation, all she has to do is open and close her legs.

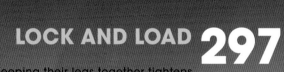

LOCK AND LOAD 297

Keeping their legs together tightens
the grip and boosts the sensations for
both partners — ready, aim, fire!

298 MAN TRAP

His pointing device naturally finds all of her pleasure spots in this pose, so she'll want to give him complete and total access to her love snare by sitting hard and clenching her groin.

UP AGAINST THE WALL **299**

Sitting while he stands lets her use her whole body to move her mouth back and forth on him without tiring out her neck.

300 MISSIONARY

Call this one the sexual equivalent of a favorite pair of old jeans — comfortable, familiar and easy to dress up or down. Even a simple act like squeezing their pelvic muscles as they push in and out turns this pose red-hot.

THE CRANKSHAFT 301

While they may not be able to keep their motors running all night in this tricky pose, her turbocharged front-to-back, side-to-side, and up-and-down driving guarantees they'll both explode before her engine blows.

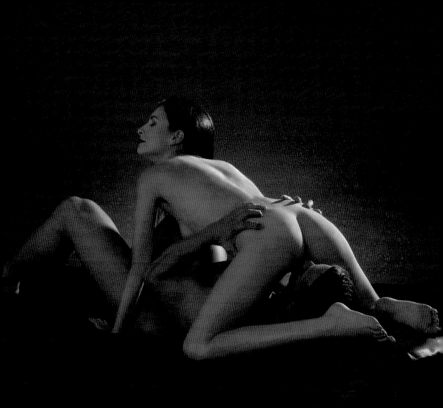

302 68 HER

Instead of trying to do two things at once, in this almost-but-not-quite 69, she can teasingly watch his excitement grow while being entirely caught up in her own blissfest.

DEEP IMPACT 303

This athletic reverse rear entry creates plenty of scope for him to move deliberately, slowly, and to the exact depth she enjoys (until his legs give out!).

304 LEANING TOWER

In this pose, he'll get off on being the king of her world while she'll get a head rush — literally. The blood racing from her pelvis to her head heightens his thrusts, creating deliciously dizzying sensations.

69 BACK 305

The bottom isn't the wrong hole. It's actually packed with sensitive nerves just begging for a good licking. By pulling her legs back during classic 69, he has full access to her backfield.

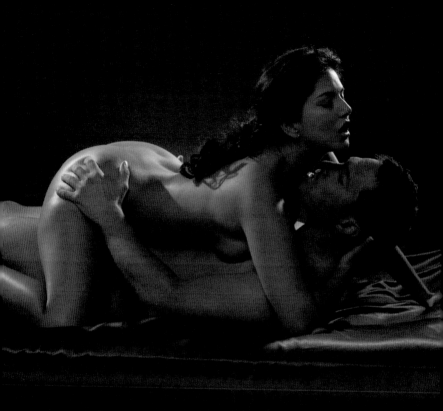

306 RUB DOWN

Forget the spa! She can treat herself to an erotic massage just by pushing up and down against his body. When she's ready for more then a rub, they don't even need to change positions.

THE STRADDLE 307

This extremely creative and somewhat challenging seated move rewards her with wonderful friction as he pushes her up against the back of the chair.

308 HANDY 69

Trying for mutual orgasms is fine, but it's not a problem if one partner's O makes an early curtain call. It will raise the excitement for the second partner, who will soon be applauding even louder and yelling for an encore.

THE SITTING CAT 309

This version of the CAT will snuggle their
pelvises together in a way sure to make
them both yowl with pleasure, and the
extra exposure means that she can also
work in some extra purr-fect strokes.

310 HOT AND SPICY

Spicing things up by adding a few naughty
moves of her own — a single leg lift and a butt
squeeze — to classic man-on-top will get his
groin doing a salsa on her most sizzling spots.

THE X FACTOR 311

The downward angle of his equipment in this pose will keep wonderful pressure on her front wall, but he may need to keep a handle on things to make sure everything stays in place.

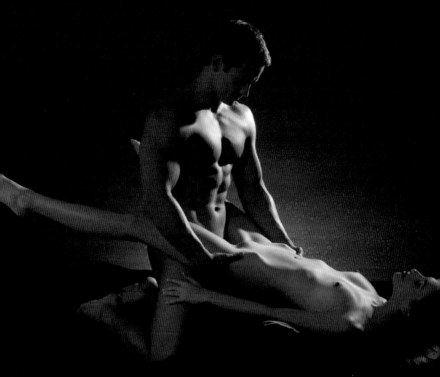

312 FIGHTER PLANE

She can lean back on a pillow for support
and let him do all the work, moving her
hips to grind her love bits against his pelvis
as he takes her in for a bumpy landing.

BE SEATED AND BESOTTED 313

This easiest of chair positions leaves each of
their hands free for the ideal opportunity to
titillate each other's pleasure-receptive nipples.

314 THE BICYCLIST

The connection between both partners will be oh-so-intimate as she opens herself up to being completely exposed to his penetrating gaze.

THE VIBE 315

Using a vibrator will definitely amp up the action, but he shouldn't limit the buzz to her love triangle. Working up and down the ultraresponsive nerves on her inner thighs will keep things humming along nicely.

316 DUET

Unlike typical rear-entry action that can leave both partners feeling disconnected, pelvises, thighs and hands touch here, making this move much more intimate and sensual.

ANYTHING GOES 317

It's hard to find a way for him to gain rear entry while still making eye contact with her. In this pose, he can look to see if her eyes are saying "yes" to some anal play before entering through her back door.

318 LOVE PUMP

Working his legs like passion levers,
she can raise them high to get some
power on the front region of her pelvis or
lower them to work her back patch.

THE PANORAMA 319

Men will loooove the eye candy that this all-access position offers. Watching her breasts bounce as she jiggles her hips is like a favorite scene out of a (high-quality) porn movie coming to life.

320 KISSING THE PINK

Most men do wrong by her when it comes to oral sex because they go for a head-on tongue-kneading. Keeping him a bit at bay and having him stick to light kisses and side licks will produce a sweeter result.

THE ACROBAT 321

Balance is definitely required for this
high-flying pose, and a safety net may
also help for postorgasmic plunges.

322 THE BIG BOUNCE

Using a stability ball as a love prop can produce body-rockin' sensations. With him sitting tight, she can bebop her hips with wild abandon, adding a slinky spring to their ultimate send-off.

LAY, LADY, LAY **323**

Despite the lack of eye contact, making
nooky doesn't get much more up-close and
personal than this. Since they're so close,
he can use her front or rear door to visit.

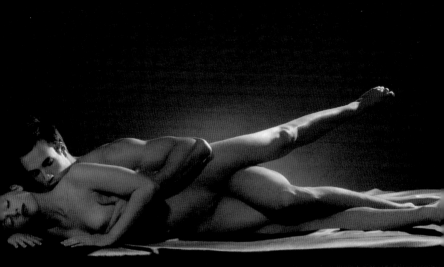

324 BENT SPOON

This is a nice middle-of-the-night pose for adding some spice to their dreams. It's easy for him to slide his leg in between hers as they spoon together in bed and enjoy a dozy cuddle.

HAPPY HANDS 325

If she is left longing after the actual deed is
done, he shouldn't be shy about fulfilling her
cravings with a little hands-on attention.

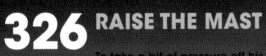

326 RAISE THE MAST

To take a bit of pressure off his pelvis, she
can lean slightly forward on her thighs — he
won't complain if her hands just happen
to slip down onto his lower deck.

UPWARD DOG **327**

With a slight arch of her back, the basic
shaggy-dog pose becomes something
to really howl with pleasure about as he
pushes against the ultrasensitive front
wall of her vagina with every stroke.

328 THE HEADLOCK

He better do everything she says and fulfill her every desire once they get in this pose, otherwise there's no telling when he will be allowed out of her leg-and-arm wrap.

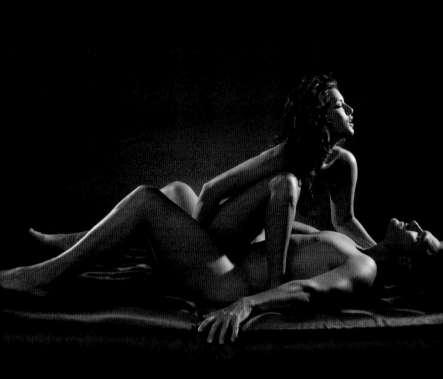

APHRODITE'S DELIGHT 329

Many women get performance jitters over the
thought of giving a helping hand during sex,
when in fact the sight of her adding fuel to their
bonfire is a surefire way to burn him up with lust.

330 STAND AND DELIVER

There isn't much for him to do in this pose but lean back, hold her up, and deliver the goods. The sexy spin for her is that she can pump her legs against the wall to get him to visit all of her pleasure spots.

DIRTY DOGGY **331**

This angle puts him in a great spot to kiss ass. If he further needs to supplicate himself, he can slide his hands between her legs and make her beg for mercy.

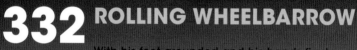

332 ROLLING WHEELBARROW

With his feet grounded and his hands firmly
holding her, this is one of the most stable
of ball positions and thus lends itself nicely
to all sorts of hot hip-hip-hoorays — shakes,
circles, rolls, thrusts, and much more.

HIGH IN THE SADDLE 333

She's angled just so to give her hot spot the direct contact it craves. To add to her pleasure party, he can double up on the stimulation by slipping his hand in between her thighs.

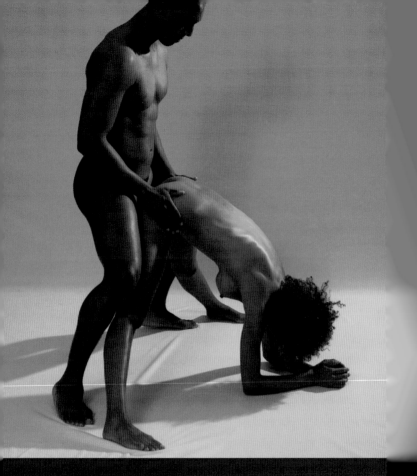

334 HEAD BENDER

This is an athletic position that requires him to have very strong legs. Spreading her legs will give him better access, but only if he can hold a knee bend that lowers him down to her entry point.

FLYING MISSIONARY 335

The limited thrusting power of this pose
is compensated by the very deliciously
direct and deep penetration.

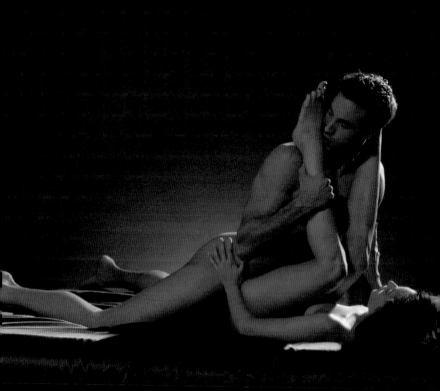

336 FOOT IN MOUTH

Giving plenty of kissing and tongue-massaging
attention to her feet during sex can be even
more orgasmic than buying a new pair of shoes.

LEAN-TO **337**

Sex from behind is usually completely in his hands — or rather, hips. But by simply hooking her legs around him, she manages a carnal conquer and takes control of the pace and depth of penetration.

338 DINING AT THE Y

Pull up a chair directly between her legs and he'll be ready for lunch at the hottest diner in town. He'll have his hands and fingers free, so he should use them to help provide pleasure across her entire plate.

TRICK OR TREAT **339**

The trick here is for him to use an up-and-down motion instead of his usual back-and-forth thrust to create some new body-to-body friction. The treat is in how sweet it will make them both feel.

340 THE ROCKER

Instead of making the common mistake of working on just that one popular spot, he can sway her hips so his tongue reaches every part of her landing strip from front to back.

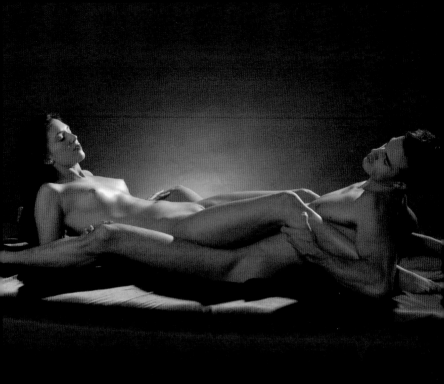

THE "X" **341**

Slow, leisurely movements will provide
enough stimulation to make up for the
lack of thrusting power in this pose.

342 EVOLVED DOG

Although not for everyone, this extremely
erotic act has him wagging her tail. When
she can't wait another second, she can
always reach down and help herself
or, of course, sit down on his bone.

ROLLER COASTER 343

This ride should make her scream with pleasure. She can heighten the thrill by closing her eyes and letting his every thrust, stroke, and touch surprise her.

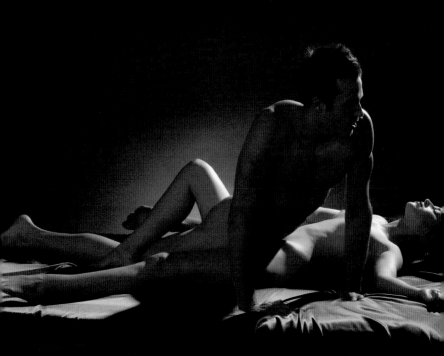

344 A LITTLE ON THE SIDE

The beauty of coming in sideways is that
he will stroke her in places not usually
reached. To max out on the pleasure, he can
alternate between wide, circular motions
and deep, up-and-down thrusting.

CRUISE CONTROL 345

He shouldn't just sit back and enjoy the ride — as much as she loves controlling the pace when she's on top, it'll feel twice as nice when he helps out by holding her hips and gently pulling her back and forth.

346 FLAMINGO

Staying in bed doesn't mean she needs to give up her favorite straddle. She won't have as much range of motion with only one leg on the ground, but this pose will still hit those familiar pleasure points.

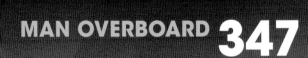

MAN OVERBOARD 347

Neither partner will have to do much in this deeply relaxing pose. To experience a wake-up burst of pleasure, she can rhythmically raise and lower her feet off the floor.

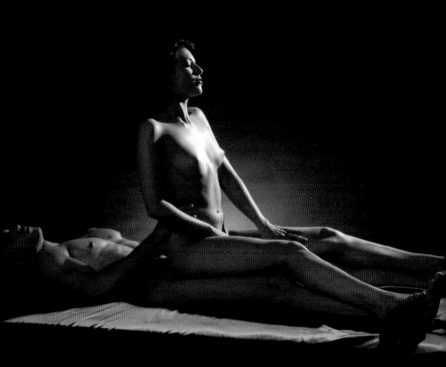

348 THE SPEED RACER

When she's in the driver's seat, it's a cinch
for her to stop rubbernecking and take
the libidinous lead so she doesn't need to
wait for him to green-light her climax.

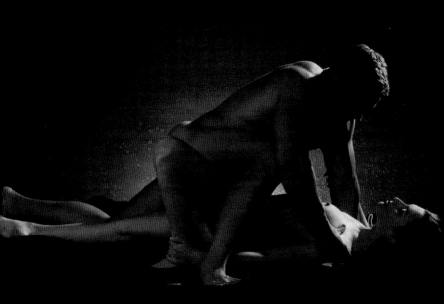

DUTCH PRETZEL **349**

They know how to add a tantalizing twist
to the action in Amsterdam. The sideways
entry means that he'll tap her hard-to-reach
spots while her upper-body bend lets them
have some intimate face-to-face action.

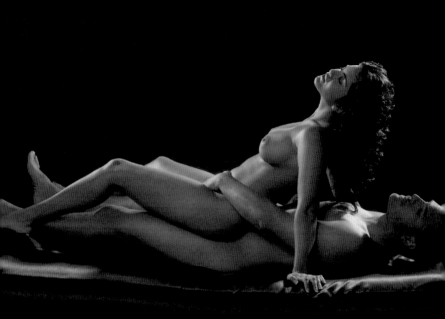

350 MANUAL CONTROL

When she lies back so that her weight is transferred to her arms, it frees him up to fiddle with her instruments, making for a very satisfying sack session (and worth the extra bicep curls she'll need to hold the pose).

G-SPOT STRIKER 351

The higher her legs, the more likely he is to bang up against her G-spot. While the ball will add an extra bounce, ultimately the stimulation of this elusive bump is only as good as the strength of his erection.

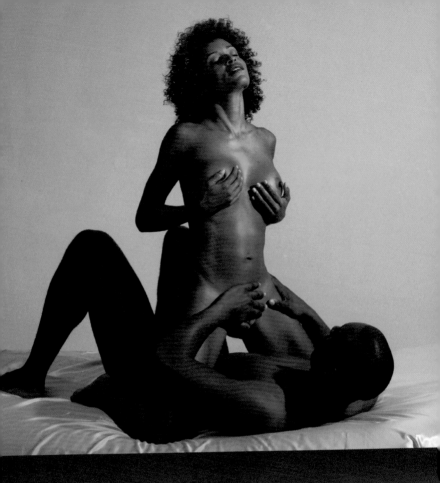

352 SPOTLIGHT

On top, in view, and out of control —
exhibitionists don't do it any other way!

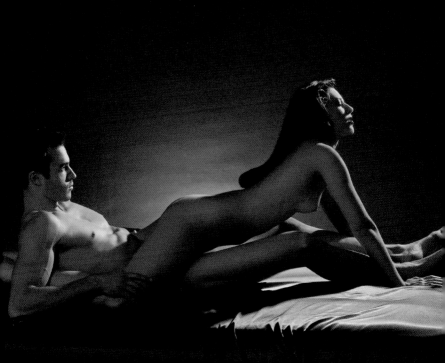

BUTTOCK DELIGHT 353

If she wants to tantalize him, she can shake
her booty ever so slightly up and down,
building him up to a rockin' orgasm.

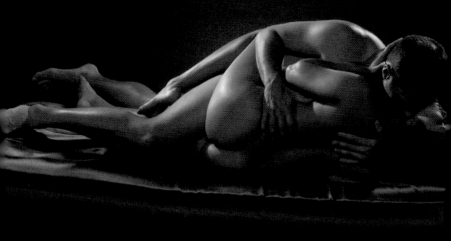

354 SOUL SIDE

What better position for two lovers in love?
Cuddling up like this is slow, romantic sex
at its best. It's a tight fit that lets them
hold each other close and sneak in lots
of kisses, nibbles and extra strokes.

FROM BALL TO WALL 355

Thanks to a little roll from the ball, she
can change her whole body's angle until
it is perfect for his penetration by simply
moving her hands up and down the wall.

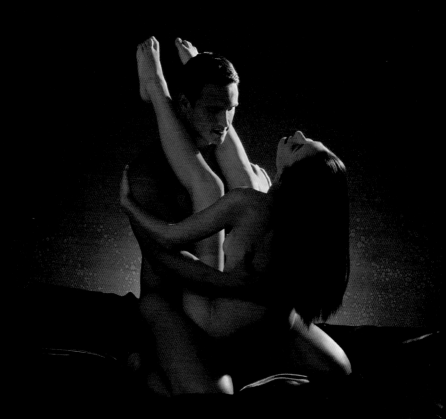

356 LEG OVER EASY

Keeping her legs tight and high will create a snugger entry for him and more sustained stimulation exactly where she needs it.

BACK BEND 357

Linger too long in this pose and she will
collapse to the floor for the wrong reason,
but the blood racing from her pelvis to
her head heightens his licks, creating
deliciously dizzying sensations that mean
she won't have to hold herself up for long.

358 REVERSE MISSIONARY

Closing her legs together makes her in charge of the action in no uncertain terms as she puts a deliciously snug squeeze on him and presses her own bliss spots at the same time.

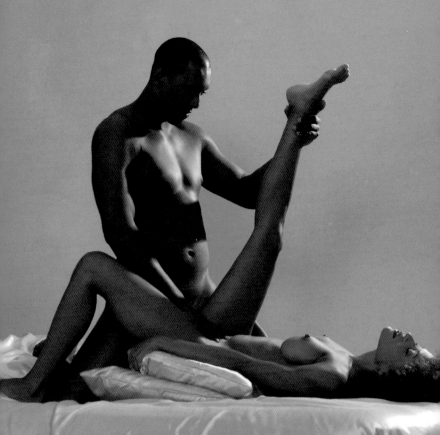

THE BUTTER CHURN 359

The slow, comfortable squeeze he'll feel as he moves her leg back and forth, combined with the extra stimulation she'll receive from his hand, will make this a steamy shoo-in for both of them.

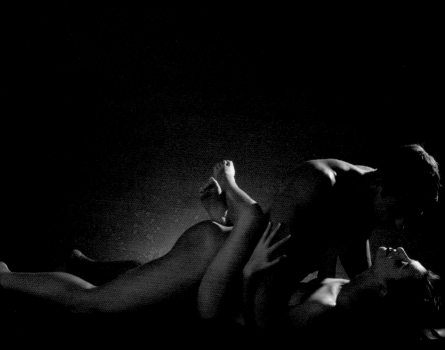

360 THE DRIVER

She may be on the bottom, but she's
in charge — by lifting her pelvis, the
speed and timing of his every thrust are
at the mercy of her wanton whims.

CANNONBALL **361**

Gravity helps them make this advanced
position a success. And luckily, her raised
legs make it a tighter space for him to
dive into, so it won't take much motion
for them to ride the orgasmic wave.

362 POWER BALL

With his feet set wide apart and her hands firmly grounded, they have a lot of stability in this pose so they can get really ballsy and make the most of the extra bounce in their gyrations.

TILT-A-GIRL 363

He may be coming in from behind, but they
still get treated to a full-frontal view of each
other's upper bodies and passion-filled faces.

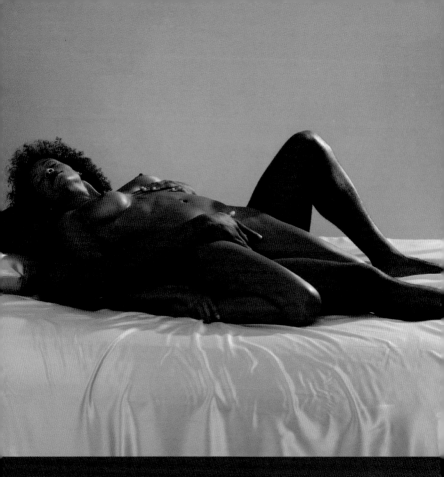

364 TRIPLE WHAMMY

With the heated combo of his leg and fingers creating friction on her nether regions and his other hand getting familiar with her breast, this move is perfectly attuned for her moaning pleasure.

TOP LOAD 365

In this one-size-fits-all pose, he can make her feel completely filled up by pressing down on her thighs once he is firmly inside of her. He won't mind the sensation of her breasts mashing up against his chest, either.

POSITIONS INDEX

366

367

368

370

371

ABOUT THE AUTHOR

Lisa Sweet is the author of numerous sexual instruction books and has had her writing published in newspapers and magazines in the United States, the United Kingdom, France, and Australia.

A New Way to Play Every Day

In this brand-new edition of the mammoth best-selling guide (which every couple should have in the bedroom), author Lisa Sweet offers tantalizing ways to spice up intimacy in and out of the bedroom. Open *365 Sex Positions* to any page and discover a sizzling new way to play together with positions like:

DRIVER'S SEAT   **OVER THE EDGE**

LONDON BRIDGE   **HEAD RUSH**

EASY RIDER   **...AND 360 MORE!!**

With stunning, tasteful, full-color photography and a range of positions from familiarly comfortable to dazzlingly acrobatic, *365 Sex Positions* has just the ideas to satisfy you both any day of the year. So why are you still reading this back cover? The fun starts inside!

ISBN-13: 978-1-64604-033-9

51995

9 781646 040339

$19.95 US
$26.95 CAN

Amorata Press